The Complete Idiot's Reference Card

The Six Guiding Principles

➤ Control
➤ Concentration
➤ Centering
➤ Focus
➤ Precision
➤ Breathing

The Apparatus Developed by Joseph Pilates

Here are the basic pieces of Pilates equipment in current use:

➤ The *Mat* bench sits several inches off the floor and includes both a strap to anchor the feet and a hand bar; it's used for the sequence of floor exercises developed by Joseph Pilates that strengthen and stretch the body and align the spine.

➤ The *Universal Reformer* is the most popular apparatus and is used to provide a total-body workout by using springs as resistance; it's a bedlike apparatus that sits low to the floor and looks like a door frame.

➤ The *Cadillac* is a bed-like table that has several springs and a trapeze suspended from the top so that you can do full body moves.

➤ The *Wunda Chair* is an advanced apparatus that works the body in motion, giving it a total-body workout; it helps develop strength, control, coordination, and balance in the body.

➤ The *Ladder Barrel* is a padded apparatus that looks like a barrel and is used mostly to stretch and strengthen the spine.

➤ The *Spine Corrector* is a lightweight padded apparatus that looks like a small barrel and is used to work the abdominals and correct posture.

➤ The *Magic Circle* is a padded low-resistance apparatus that looks like a circle and is used to work the inner thighs and arm muscles.

tear here

alpha
books

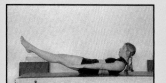

The Hundred

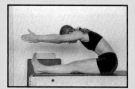

Roll-Up

Leg Circles

Rolling Like a Ball

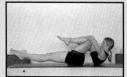

Single-Leg Stretch

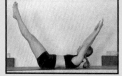

Double-Leg Stretch

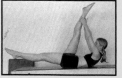

Single Straight-Leg Stretch

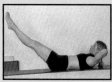

Double Straight-Leg Stretch

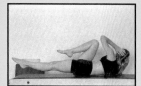

Crisscross

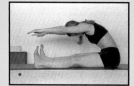

Spine Stretch

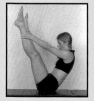

Open-Leg Rocker

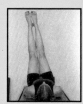

Corkscrew 1

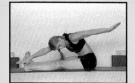

The Saw

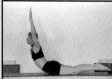

Swan Dive

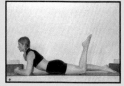

Single-Leg Kick

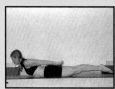

Double-Leg Kick

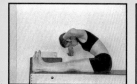

Neck Pull

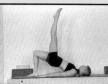

Shoulder Bridge

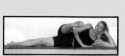

Side-Kick Series

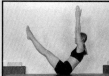

Teaser 3

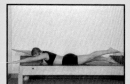

Swimming

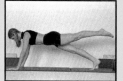

Leg Pull Front

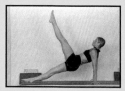

Leg Pull Back

The Seal

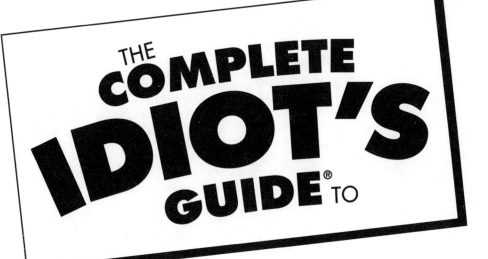

THE COMPLETE IDIOT'S GUIDE® TO

the Pilates Method

by Karon Karter

alpha books

201 West 103rd Street
Indianapolis, IN 46290

A Pearson Education Company

This book is dedicated to my devoted mother, who I love more than life itself, and Janet Harris, my writing coach, who continues to mold and shape my writing career.

Copyright © 2001 by Karon Karter

International Standard Book Number: 0-02-863983-9
Library of Congress Catalog Card Number: Available upon request.

03   02   01   8   7   6   5   4   3   2

Interpretation of the printing code: The rightmost number of the first series of numbers is the year of the book's printing; the rightmost number of the second series of numbers is the number of the book's printing. For example, a printing code of 01-1 shows that the first printing occurred in 2001.

Printed in the United States of America

Note: This publication contains the opinions and ideas of its author. It is intended to provide helpful and informative material on the subject matter covered. It is sold with the understanding that the author and publisher are not engaged in rendering professional services in the book. If the reader requires personal assistance or advice, a competent professional should be consulted.

Publisher
Marie Butler-Knight

Product Manager
Phil Kitchel

Managing Editor
Cari Luna

Senior Acquisitions Editor
Randy Ladenheim-Gil

Development Editor
Michael Koch

Production Editor
JoAnna Kremer

Copy Editor
Krista Hansing

Illustrator
Jody P. Schaeffer

Cover Designers
Mike Freeland
Kevin Spear

Book Designers
Scott Cook and Amy Adams of DesignLab

Indexer
Angie Bess

Layout/Proofreading
Angela Calvert
Mary Hunt

Contents at a Glance

Part 1: Live in Your Body   **1**

  1 Join the Movement   3
Learn how Pilates works hand in hand with your real life and find a whole new way to get your body moving.

  2 Fix Your Frame   19
Find out how Pilates can improve your posture. One of the hallmarks of Pilates is that it can alleviate most back pain.

  3 Take Your Breath   33
Discover how your breath can enhance your life.

  4 (Re)Discover the Perfect Body   45
Find out what the Pilates method can do for you and how to train yourself right.

Part 2: Show Me the Mat   **55**

  5 Befriend Your Body   57
Joseph Pilates understood the secret to attaining poise and grace. You need to work the body from within—every muscle evenly, no matter how small.

  6 Sculpt Yourself into Shape   73
Now you're ready to tackle the Mat workout. Follow the introductory exercises in this chapter, and you're off to a great start.

  7 Get the Man-Made Mat Body   89
Great bodies are made, not born. It's the exercises in this chapter that give you body results. You, too, can obtain the man-made body.

  8 Graduate to the "It" Body   103
Love-handle free and loving life. Add seven new exercises to your Mat routine to chisel your body so that you can flaunt it.

Part 3: Moving On Up   **117**

  9 Smart Sweating   119
It's time to sweat! Put an edge on the introductory work. You'll add several advanced Mat exercises that turn the heat way up.

10 The Intelligent Workout 135

As you complete the Mat finish line, you'll find out why your brain, along with your muscles, is challenged to the max.

11 The Anticellulite Solution 151

Shouldn't those dimples be reserved for your face cheeks? You can tighten those areas that seem to travel south with the Side-Kick Series in this chapter.

12 Flexing Muscles 165

Whittle away the flabby skin that waddles long after you've lifted your arm to wave hello. With the Standing Arms Series in this chapter, you'll be saying hello to slender, defined arms.

Part 4: Instruments of Torture **179**

13 Body Reformer: The Rack 181

You'll wiggle into a weird-looking medieval device, wrap your toes around a bar, hold on to a pair of leather handles, and pull back and forth on a bed-like platform. This chapter introduces you to the beginning Universal Reformer workout.

14 Bednasium: The Cadillac 197

Find out about the variety of full-body moves that you can do with the Cadillac, a medieval-looking bed with springs and a trapeze. These moves bring you back to the days of hanging off a swing set.

15 Body in Motion: The Wunda Chair 211

It does "Wunders" for your body. You need more than strength to tackle the exercises on the Wunda Chair. Joseph Pilates said, "Everyone needs one in his living room."

16 Spinal Soother: The Barrels 221

Joseph Pilates said, "You're as old as your spine is flexible." In this chapter, you'll see a few exercises that leave you feeling oh-so-stretched!

17 Simply Fit: The Magic Circle 231

You prefer to exercise at home. Besides convenient, it's prudent. Enter the Magic Circle, another Joseph Pilates invention.

Part 5: Forever Fit   **243**

   18 The Art of Teaching   245
      Find out if you have what it takes to join the Pilates
      movement.

   19 If You Build It, They Will Come   257
      Don't just sculpt your butt—save it. Why not open up a
      Pilates gym? Learn how to get started and make a good
      living while teaching your passion, Pilates.

   20 The Many Faces of Joseph Pilates   269
      For years master teachers have passed on Joseph Pilates's
      work. Find out what style is right for you.

Appendixes

   A Certification Programs   279
   B Glossary   281
     Index   285

Contents

Part 1: Live in Your Body   **1**

1   Join the Movement   **3**

Introducing the Pilates Method 3
The Thinking Body 5
Body Therapy 6
The Man Behind the Method 7
Your Inner Athlete 8
The Achy Breaky Body 9
Granny Got Her Groove Back 10
Stay Stronger Longer 10
Battling Brittle Bones 11
A Pea in a Pod 12
   Is It for You? 12
   Listen to the Doctor's Orders 13
In the Pursuit of Excellence 14
Sweat Isn't Enough 14
Strength and Length 15
Risky Business 16
Shattered Dreams 17
A New You 17

2   Fix Your Frame   **19**

Message in Your Body 19
Torso Talk 20
No More Pain in the Back 21
How Are Your Curves? 23
Got a Slumper, Here! 23
   What's Up with Your Shoulders? 24
   Is Your Head Straight? 25
Too Much Arch in Your Back 25
   Putting Your Pelvis in Neutral 26
   Supplying Spine Support 28
The Powerhouse 29
Where's Your Body? 30

3   Take Your Breath   **33**

With Every Breath You Take 33
   Breathe Like a Baby 35
   Discover Your Basic Breath 35
Detoxify Your Body 37
Work on Your Stamina 39

Become a Better Breather 40
The Rules: Breathe Right! 41
Avoid Running On Empty 42
Let It Flow 42
Vow to Get More Air 42
Trust Your Nose 43
Tune Up Your Breath 43

4 (Re)Discover the Perfect Body   **45**

Spring to Life 45
The Art of Training 46
Concentrate on Your Moves 46
Control is Crucial 46
Discover Your Center 47
Find Your Flow 47
Move with Precision 47
Build Your Breath 48
Metabolism Makeover 48
Train Yourself to a Better Body 48
Eat Yourself Healthy 49
Train Yourself Right—in Six Weeks 50
Away with Aerobics? No Way! 51
The Not-So-New Fitness 51
Body Beautiful, but Not in a Day! 52

Part 2: Show Me the Mat   **55**

5 Befriend Your Body   **57**

Body Wisdom 58
Training with Symmetry: Muscle Imbalances 59
Your Cheating Body 60
Checking Out Your Form 61
Initiation: Learning the Concepts 61
Learning the Lingo: Pre-Pilates 62
Transforming Your Transverse: Scoop 62
Spine to Mat 64
Peel Your Spine off the Mat 64
Propelling Your Pelvis: Pelvic Clock Work 66
Chin to Your Chest 67
Pits to Your Hips 68
Pinch, Pinch, Pinch Your Butt Cheeks 70
Pinch, Lift, and Grow Tall 70
Just for Feet 71
Before You Go! 71

6   Sculpt Yourself into Shape   73

A Perfect 10 73
Strike a Stance: The Pilates "V" 74
Wake Up Your Body with the Hundred 75
Roll-Up 77
Flex and Stretch: Hamstrings, Ankles, Leg Circles 78
  Ankle Circles 79
  Leg Circles 79
Rolling Like a Ball 80
Single- and Double-Leg Stretch 81
  Single-Leg Stretch 82
  Double-Leg Stretch 83
Spine Stretch 84
The Saw 84
Seal 86
Wrapping It Up 86

7   Get the Man-Made Mat Body   89

Busting Your Gut 89
  Securing Your Scoop 90
  The Strong and Long 91
Corkscrews, Swans, and Neck Pulls, Oh My! 92
Open-Leg Rocker 93
The Corkscrew 94
Take Flight with the Swan 95
Single-Leg Kick 97
The Much-Needed Rest: Child's Pose 99
Back to the Belly: Neck Pull 99
It's a Wrap 101

8   Graduate to the "It" Body   103

Flaunting Your Flow 103
Ready, Set, Rhythm? 104
If You've Got It, Flaunt It! 105
Love-Handle-Free and Loving It: The Fives 106
Double-Leg Kick 109
Shoulder Bridge (Stability) 110
Teaser 1 111
Let's Go Swimming 112
Head to Heel Like Steel: Leg Pulls 113
The Finish Line 115

Part 3: Moving On Up   117

9 Smart Sweating   119

Boosting Your Ability 120
Tackling the Next Level 121
What's Next? 121
Control Is Crucial: The Rollover 122
Hush Your Hips: Shoulder Bridge with Kicks 124
It's a Stretch: Spine Twist 125
Straight as a Pencil: The Jackknife 126
Just Not Any Only Old Teaser: Super-Advanced 128
Head to Heel Like Steel: Leg Pulls and Push-Ups 129
Going the Other Way: Leg Pull Back 130
A Different Class of Push-Up 130
Be the Boss of Your Body 133

10 The Intelligent Workout   135

Body and Mind Integration 135
See It, and Then Do It! 137
The Swan Dive 138
Age-Defying Moves: The Scissors and the Bicycle 139
Let's Dance: Can-Can to Hip Circles 141
Hip Circles 142
Precision Lifts: Kneeling Side Kicks, the Mermaid,
   and the Twist 143
Pure Stretch: The Mermaid *145*
The Twist *145*
Balance in Motion: The Boomerang 147
Last Call 149

11 The Anticellulite Solution   151

De-Fat Your Dimples 151
Empowering Your Patootie 152
Stay Square 153
Off to Get a Better Butt: Weeks 1 and 2 154
Bye, Bye, Butt Rut: Weeks 3 and 4 156
Giving Up Your Rear: Weeks 5 and 6 160
Boosting Your Bottom Line 164

12 Flexing Muscles   165

To Tense or Not to Tense 166
My Stiff Neck 167
Muscle, Not Momentum! 167
Leaning into the Wind 168

Jiggy-Free: The Standing Arms Series 169
Basic Biceps 170
Boxing 171
Develop Your Delts 172
Pump It Up: Zip-Ups 173
Stretch, Flex, Go: Circles, Chest Expansion, and Side Stretch 174
Minor But Mighty 177

Part 4: Instruments of Torture   **179**

13   Body Reformer: The Rack   **181**

The Rack: Reform It! 181
No Weights, No Problem! 182
Who Needs a Reformer? 182
The Underworked Muscles: The Feet 183
The Total Body Reformer Workout 185
Starting Off: The Foot Work 186
The Hundred 188
Leg Circles 190
The Stomach Massage Series 190
Short Box Series 192
Knee Stretches 194
Take a Run: Running 195
Just Right! 196

14   Bednasium: The Cadillac   **197**

Cruising Your Cadillac 197
Aimless It Ain't! 198
No Short Cuts! 199
Cadillac Classics: The Exercises 200
Returning to Core Concept: Rolling Back 201
Breathe Right! Breathing 201
Oh La La: The Leg Spring Series 203
The Monkey 207
Hanging Up 208
Half-Hang 209
This Bed Is for You 209

15   Body in Motion: The Wunda Chair   **211**

It Does "Wunders" for Your Body 211
Balance in Motion: Wunda Chair Basics 212
Washer Woman 214
The Pike 214
Stretch with Pumping 216

xi

Swan on the Floor 216
The Jackknife 217
Spine Stretch 218
Body Talk 219

16 Spinal Soother: The Barrels   **221**

Big and Small: The Barrels 221
Baby Your Body 222
Moving in Place: Basic Barrel Moves 223
Gittyap: Horseback 224
Backward Stretch 225
Low Barrel Moves: Exercises 226
The Scissors, the Bicycle, and Rolling In and Out 226
Stretch Over the Barrel with Arm Circles 229
Baby Your Back 230

17 Simply Fit: The Magic Circle   **231**

Introducing the Big O 231
Work It with the Big O 232
Gut Buster 233
Upper Body De-jiggle with the Magic Circle 234
Lower-Body Buster with the Big O 235
With Your Back Against a Wall 237
Working the Wall 238
Slide Down the Wall 238
Rolling Down the Wall 240
The End 241

Part 5: Forever Fit   **243**

18 The Art of Teaching   **245**

Give Life to a 90-Year-Old Method 246
Aiming for Excellence 246
Get to Know the Clients 247
Made to Order: Program Designs 248
Tip-Top Training: Strategies for the Teacher 249
"F" Is for Frequency 249
"I" Is for Intensity 250
"T" Is for Time 251
Dealing with Clients 251
Keep Clients on Their Toes 251
No Poking, Pushing, or Prodding 252
Practice KISS 252
Praise for Results 253
Patience, Please 253

But I've Never Danced! 253
Stay True to the System 254
Where the Core Is! 254
Listen Up! 255
For the Love of Teaching 256

19 If You Build It, They Will Come   257

Are You a Homebody or Gym Body? 257
Just Don't Sculpt Your Bottom, Save It! 258
No Money Tree? 260
Who Are You? 261
What Are You Offering? 262
Booking Your Clients 263
The Big Bucks 263
  The A-Team 263
  Now Hiring the A-Team 263
  For Rent! 264
  Field of Dreams 265
Start Spreading the News 265
  Buying the Equipment 266
  Finding the Right Stuff? 267

20 The Many Faces of Pilates   269

The Good Old Days! 269
Will the Real Pilates Stand Up? 270
Sign Me Up to Join the Movement 272
Study the Universal Method 273
Avoid the Quacks 275
The Universal Method Is Here for Good! 275
A Growing Trend 276

Appendixes

A Certification Programs   279

B Glossary   281

Index   285

Foreword

In the early part of the twentieth century, Joseph Pilates created an exercise system that is taking the twenty-first century by storm. He called his technique "Contrology." Today, while not a household (yet) name, his method is commonly known as "Pilates."

Pilates has evolved as the generic name for unusual stretching and toning exercises, just as "aerobic" is used for the various forms of classes created for cardiovascular work. This is unfortunate. The method created by Joseph Pilates—and painstakingly handed down through his pupils—had direction, purpose, and guiding principles that are often missing today in what is called Pilates. Karon Karter's research and personal experience, coupled with her energetic writing style, embody the vitality and integrity of the classic work.

My introduction to the method came through a diluted form of the traditional work that lacked rhythm and dynamics. But just this "tinkering at the margins" was efficacious enough to inspire me to meet and study with some of the teachers who passed the work down from Joseph Pilates, enhancing my understanding of what the original work was really about. Studying with Romana Krzanowsky in New York and Houston opened my mind, my body, and my sprit to the richness and vitality of the traditional work. Exposure to Kathy Grant and Ron Fletcher, other teachers who studied with Pilates, proved equally transforming and educational. All of them left their unique imprint upon my teaching and inspired my understanding of Pilates's work.

My teaching experiences over the last two decades have brought home the utter importance of the concepts and movement techniques of the traditional work of Joseph Pilates. When mentally understood and physically performed, it affects the entire functionality of the human being in a life-enhancing manner. It changes your spirit. It changes your life. Karon Karter is to be acknowledged for her dedication to a system that will prove beneficial to generations to come. With her book, she provides a comprehensive view of the traditional, inspiring her readers to search out the magic of Joseph Pilates.

—*Colleen Glenn*
Owner and teacher instructor of the Goodbody's System Certification Program

Introduction

Rather than sucking in your gut and wishing that you looked svelte in your wetsuit, affectionately known as the little black dress, try Pilates: It's a whole torso workout that strengthens the abs and back and that also straightens your posture, making you feel taller. Pilates is the wave of the future, combining the allure of rebalancing your mind as you fine-tune from head to toe; it possesses tremendous appeal. Here's Joseph Pilates's prophecy: In 10 sessions, you'll feel the difference; in 20, you'll see the difference; in 30, you'll have a new body.

How This Book Is Organized

The book is divided into six parts. Whether you want to expand your knowledge or try Pilates for the first time, the pages in this book will be your guide. Here's a quick overview:

Part 1, "Live in Your Body," explains why you want to join the Pilates movement. As you read on, you will find out about the muscles that support your frame and keep you standing tall. Plus, you'll discover why your breath can enhance your life.

Part 2, "Show Me the Mat," introduces Mat exercises in the correct sequence and core concepts so that you can get the body that you so deserve. These exercises are the same ones taught by Joseph Pilates. Before long, you'll move just like Joseph Pilates.

Part 3, "Moving On Up," was written with two goals in mind: to challenge you and to give you enough exercises for a lifetime. In this part, you'll learn the advanced Mat exercises, plus the Side-Kick Series and the Standing Arms Series.

Part 4, "Instruments of Torture," introduces the equipment that Joseph Pilates developed more than 90 years ago: the Universal Reformer, the Cadillac, the Wunda Chair, the Electric Chair, the Ladder Barrel, the Spine Corrector, and the Magic Circle.

Part 5, "Forever Fit," explores other avenues of Pilates. For example, do you have what it takes to join the Universal Method? Or how about opening up your own studio? Many styles of Pilates are popping up in health clubs. Is that style right for you?

A Little Something Else!

This book also contains a few easy-to-recognize sidebars that offer inspirational quotes from Joseph Pilates, as well as tips, lingo, and extra information to help you along the way. Keep an eye out for the following elements to enhance your knowledge:

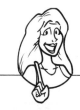

Pilates Lingo

These boxes contain words or common lingo used in Pilates. Lengthen your lingo, and you're on your way to perfecting your Pilates.

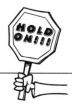

Pilates Precaution

These boxes contain warnings for the students to prevent them from getting into a sticky situation.

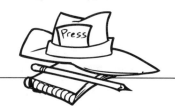

Pilates Scoop

These boxes contain tips and tidbits about Pilates that may be helpful while you practice this method.

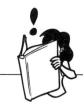

Pilates Primer

These boxes contain inspirational quotes from Joseph Pilates, along with historical information.

Acknowledgments

Yes, I dreamed it and put my thoughts to words to invent this book. However, this enormous task couldn't have been accomplished without so many gracious people.

A very special thanks to Toni Beck, the 50-plus coordinator and researcher for the Baylor/Tom Landry Sports Medicine and Research Center in Dallas, Texas. She defies her age with grace and beauty.

A thank-you debt that I'll never be able to return extends to my graphic designer, Bo Mikolajczyk. He stayed up with me all night to design the pictures for this book the way I wanted them.

Thank you to *City Lights of San Francisco,* my favorite workout clothes, for providing me with some great-looking outfits for the pictures in this book. And a special thanks goes to Kristin Moses (she just had a baby six months prior to the shoot and looks great—thanks to Pilates) for modeling and allowing me to shoot the pictures in this book in her studio, Perform Studio.

Hugs and kisses to MGB—thank you for your emotional support and patience during the months of this project.

I'm grateful for the entire team at Alpha Books, especially Michael Koch and JoAnna Kremer, who massaged my words even more to make this a great book—this is our second book together and I just love their work. Of course, I wouldn't have a book if my editor, Randy Ladenheim-Gil, didn't like my idea of this book. So, many thanks for keeping me moving toward my passion.

My family is great, because they continue to support me during the ups and downs of my writing career.

I can't leave without giving Colleen Glenn a special thank you. She taught me Pilates; her certification program is the best one out there! But that's not all. Thank you so much for your emotional support and for sharing your expertise with me while I wrote this book.

Trademarks

All terms mentioned in this book that are known to be or are suspected of being trademarks or service marks have been appropriately capitalized. Alpha Books and Pearson Education cannot attest to the accuracy of this information. Use of a term in this book should not be regarded as affecting the validity of any trademark or service mark.

Part 1

Live in Your Body

This part introduces you to your frame and the muscles that support your "center" and keep you standing tall. You'll also learn about your breath and how good breathing techniques enhance your life. In short, this part gets you ready for the chapters to come and helps you heighten your life for the better.

Chapter 1

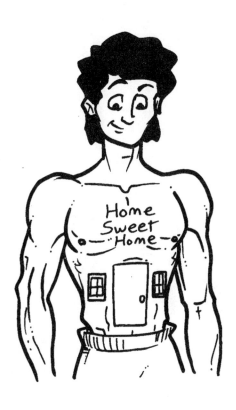

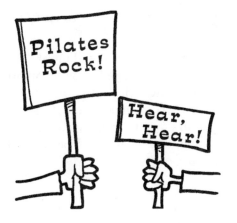

Join the Movement

In this Chapter

➤ Introducing the Pilates method

➤ The thinking body

➤ The man behind the method

➤ Stay stronger longer

➤ A discipline for all walks of life

Would you believe me if I told you there is a workout that can give you longer, leaner legs and buns to die for without weight-room bulk? What if I told you also that this same workout gives you a firmer, flatter midsection and improves your posture, and that it can also make you taller and feel energized and challenged? Would you still believe me? Now, imagine the unthinkable: You actually look forward to this workout.

Introducing the Pilates Method

Joseph Pilates (1880–1967), pronounced "puh-LAH-teez," is the visionary behind this promising workout. The Pilates method is a total body-conditioning workout for both men and women that engages you and leaves you refreshed and alert with an enormous amount of self-confidence. It's an intense, ongoing challenge blending Eastern and Western philosophies of physical and mental conditioning.

The Pilates method gives you the stretching benefits of a yoga class along with the great muscle tone of a nautilus workout. This discipline focuses on muscular harmony and balance; it's a whole new way to get your body moving. But don't take my word for it—see what others have to say.

Here are some testimonies from students of mine, who share their reasons for taking and loving it; see where you fit in:

"After participating in a Mat class for less than a year, I have found my abdominal muscles to be stronger than in any other form of exercise I've done for more than 20 years. Because of this abdominal toning paired with very concentrated and controlled breathing patterns, my spine has become much more flexible and my posture more erect. Pilates has helped improve the quality of other forms of exercise such as Yoga and weight lifting. I only wish I had begun studying it years ago."

—Sandra Roberdeau

"What Pilates has done for me is elongate my muscles; I look leaner just by using my own body weight for resistance. I do so many other forms of exercise—kickboxing, running, aerobics, spinning, and weight training. However, with Pilates, I feel I am getting just as much of a 'workout' and am being gentler and kinder to myself. And I do the Mat exercises right in my hotel room while I travel for my job, which I do half the month."

—Penny Pollack

"I am a 60-year old woman and former health club owner who has worked out almost daily for the last 20 years. I had been doing some form of cardio workout daily, combined with weight training with a personal trainer twice a week and a twice-weekly yoga class. For the past few years, I had not seen much gain in strength or loss of weight, until I began taking a Pilates Mat class. My body has responded to this new discipline. My muscles feel longer and stronger, and even though I have not lost any weight, I am trimmer. These classes are also a work out for the mind—you have to concentrate on what you are doing."

—Terry Casey

Pilates Primer

In the words of Joseph Pilates, "The Prophecy: In 10 sessions, you'll feel the difference; in 20, you'll see the difference; and in 30, you'll have a whole new body."

"Pilates is an escape for me from the daily rush. It is the only time of the day that I concentrate on myself. I always feel good for the rest of the day after a class and actually feel taller! Having three children (twins and two C-sections), I look forward to my classes with Karon for both mental and physical conditioning."

—Wendy Poston

"After two back surgeries, my physical therapist recommended Pilates. I have been exercising with the Mat for over a year now, and my back feels great."

"In fact, my posture is better, I feel taller, and I am more flexible and stronger that ever. By strengthening those 'core' muscles, the stabilizing muscles, I am able to do everything I did before back problems, and do them better."

—Kurt Liese

The Pilates workout changes how you feel about your own body. It increases your vitality, makes you feel years younger, and improves your posture while toning those "flabby" muscles. Furthermore, the Pilates system eliminates most nagging back pain, and your sex life will improve because you will function better in those vital areas. Plus, you'll love your body.

The Thinking Body

Pilates creates a thinking body. I'm sure you're familiar with the five senses—sight, smell, hearing, taste, and touch. But we also get information from various inner senses that make up our *proprioceptive* system, which literally means "own reception." This system is sort of an internal dialogue that feeds us information: to eat, to drink, to stop, to go. Deep within us, this system communicates information about our own bodies that no one else is privy to. Proprioception coordinates our every movement in time and space; it enables the pianist to place his fingers in the right place without looking or the quarterback to know instinctively when to take the ball and run with it. Our mind has an innate way to control our muscles so that they perform what we want.

The exercises designed by Joseph Pilates require concentration and precision of movement. With practice and repetition, you'll fine-tune your proprioceptive sense and learn to focus mentally. Eventually, your body will execute these moves, no matter how demanding, with precision, control, and fluidity of motion without having to think about what you're doing.

To be sure, some exercises are difficult. Your legs may quake and you may hear that voice in your

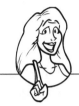

Pilates Lingo

Proprioceptive system literally means "own reception." Proprioception coordinates every movement in time and space; it enables the pianist to place his fingers in the right place without looking or the quarterback to know instinctively when to take the ball and run with it. These exercises are designed to get you to know your body.

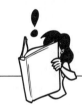

Pilates Primer

Joseph Pilates called his method "Contrology" because it was designed to teach exercisers how to gain the mastery of their minds over the compete control of their bodies.

5

head: "Give up. This is too hard." Don't listen! These moves pinpoint imbalances in your body, whether it's lack of strength, coordination, flexibility, balance, or muscular imbalances. Everyone has weaknesses, but with practice and repetition, these moves get easier as your mind tells your body what to do. Accomplishing this feat proves to you that you can do more for yourself—and your life. Pushing yourself when you think "I can't" is a gift to yourself—that's empowering.

Perseverance stays with you long after the workout. You'll learn to live in your body and have a certain level of awareness about yourself. You'll learn to embrace its imbalances, find ways to overcome them, accept yourself a little better, and like your body a little more because you didn't give up—that's self-discipline.

When you're mentally in tune with what you're doing, you become physically alert; the mind controls the body. These exercises can help you achieve this heightened level of well-being—to live in your body.

Pilates Scoop

Self-discipline means regulating oneself for the sake of self-improvement, which is what Joseph Pilates espoused and embodied!

Body Therapy

Thanks to the era of the couch potato, we've witnessed a dramatic shift in our bodies. It's gone south, right? Yet, it's not too late to get your body in motion. This immobility ruins your bodies. Besides flabby muscles, movement in your joints becomes rusty.

To stop this decay, we need to strengthen and stretch your bodies. We all know that there are no shortcuts to a better body, so we must get our bottoms off the couch. How about learning to use your body, but not in an out-of-breath, heart-pounding sweat session?

The exercises in this book are more subtle. As you grow with movement, you'll learn things about your body, particularly its imbalances. You'll also learn how to listen to your body—you know, those subtle aches and pains and hidden quirks.

Ever get frustrated because you can't do what you used to do at 20? With a little more wear and tear on our bodies, most of us can't move like we used to. We get tighter as we age. Is that so bad, though? If we didn't grow older, then we would stay stagnant, emotionally and physically. Pilates teaches you to grow; an aging body doesn't have to deteriorate.

Embrace your weaknesses so that you'll learn how to live in harmony with your body, young or old. Joseph Pilates's methods, in a sense, keep you moving forward.

Do you live with chronic pain, perhaps a stiff lower back, a popping knee, or an achy shoulder? You live with these hidden stresses every day. Your body has learned to cope with them. Many students claim that only after training in Pilates had they realized that they've been living with chronic pain. For example, minor back pains. Have you ever stopped to think why your back aches? Could it be from movements that you take for granted?

Your everyday movements might take a toll on your body. Instead of moving through life in an out-of-control, jerky manner, use Joseph's methods, which teach controlled moves and no traumatic movements. This control will spill over into your everyday life. As you become more aware of your body and how it functions, you are more likely to live a healthier life.

With these exercises, you'll increase flexibility, improve balance and coordination, build strength, and tone muscles; it's a resistance workout without all that bulk. These exercises can also help you improve your posture, rejuvenate your energy level, relieve stress, and reduce fatigue and chronic pain. Within every exercise, you'll work on the following:

➤ Flexibility

➤ Strength

➤ Balance

➤ Coordination

The exercises offer a complete connection between body and mind; it's a feel-great workout because you don't have to run yourself ragged to get in shape.

By accomplishing the exercises described in this book, you can take a timeout from the daily pressures of life, have a quiet session for your mind, and get rid of the body blues. You can feel good about your body as you witness a little shift in flab composition and gain a tremendous amount of self-confidence—and, in doing so, you'll create a new happier you.

Pilates Primer

Here is Joseph Pilates's 1945 definition of the ideal physical fitness: "The attainment and maintenance of a uniformly developed body with a sound mind fully capable of naturally, easily, and satisfactorily performing our many and varied daily tasks with spontaneous zest and pleasure."

The Man Behind the Method

Joseph Pilates was a legendary body healer. His own sickly childhood made him passionate about ways to combat sickness through conditioning and strengthening the body. In fact, asthma and other childhood aliments didn't keep him from becoming an accomplished gymnast, boxer, diver, and skier.

He admired the Eastern traditions of mindful body conditioning, particularly its focus on calmness, freeing the mind and being centered and whole, with an emphasis on stretching. In addition, he mastered the Western approach to Greek and German fitness that emphasized strength and muscle tone. Joseph Pilates combined the two to develop his own mind and body workout.

Joseph Pilates had an opportunity to experiment with his principles during World War I. As a nurse, he invented exercise apparatus for the inactive patients by attaching springs to their hospital beds. He invented ways to exercise their limbs, stretch their spines, and develop their core strength while bedridden. In fact, he used anything that he could get his hands on—his bunk, the bedsprings, and a chair, for example. This inspiration was the prototype of several pieces of equipment used today. Ninety years ago, his vision was just a concept. Today, however, you'll see this equipment in most studios, plus the real heart of his work, the Mat workout.

Pilates Primer

In a 1959 interview, Joseph Pilates said, "Movements are planned to relieve the heart, lungs, and liver of constriction caused by modern day living ...."

What was amazing, given such distressed surroundings, is that his methods worked. Because Joseph was so successful at getting his patients moving, he was asked to train the most elite armed forces of the British military. After that, performers and many athletes turned to Joseph for hard-core training. For example, Max Schmelling, the famous heavyweight sensation, relied on Joseph to train him.

Of course, behind every great man, there's a woman. Clara Pilates was devoted to her husband and his work; she was a nurse who immigrated with him from Germany to live the American dream. In 1926, they opened their first studio in New York City on 939 Eighth Avenue and taught Joseph's vision of ideal fitness. The Pilates Movement is 90 years older than most traditional exercise programs.

Your Inner Athlete

Chances are you've heard of Pilates but really are not sure what to expect or even if you can do this workout. Anyone can do it; your fitness level doesn't matter. The Pilates method can be your primary mode of body conditioning and injury prevention, or you can supplement it with your own weekly exercise routine. That was Joseph's dream, a workout that can be used by everyone, from basic to advanced, from the injured to the super-fit, at any age and any level of ability.

You won't sweat to loud music, nor will you pound the pavement to achieve great muscle tone. You won't lift anything heavier than a set of 5-pound dumbbell weights.

Instead, this discipline is based on six extremely sound principles: concentration, control, centering, flow, precision, and breathing. The routines are biomechanically safe and nonimpact; the moves stretch and strengthen all the major muscle groups without neglecting the smaller, weaker muscles.

There are two ways to work your body: a group Mat class or an individually instructed lesson using the apparatus invented by Joseph Pilates. You can do both. Each Mat class was specifically designed to work your muscles in a logical sequence. Some of the names given to these moves sound more like a game of Twister—the Teaser, the Boomerang, the Rollover. And get ready for a swim; however, you won't get your toes wet. A typical Mat class lasts about an hour and costs about $10 to $20 apiece.

Don't feel panicked by the medieval-looking machines equipped with leather straps, springs, and a trapeze if you decide to train on the specially designed equipment. Keep in mind that this equipment was designed more than 90 years ago and delivers body results— an uplifted derriere, flat-ripped abs, and sleek, slender legs; it could be the only real anticellulite solution.

Joseph Pilates invented more than 500 specific exercises on these machines to develop the body uniformly: the Universal Reformer, the Cadillac, the Wunda Chair, the Electric Chair, the Spinal Corrector, Ladder Barrel, Ped-a-Pole, and the Magic Circle.

Don't fret—you won't be doing many repetitions. In other words, you won't crunch your heart out for sleek abs. Joseph Pilates preferred fewer, more precise movements, requiring proper control and form. A typical workout will last an hour and, depending on the teacher, can cost about $50 to $75 per session.

The Achy Breaky Body

The Pilates movement is now getting a fair amount of respect from the rehabilitative community. Physical therapists, chiropractors, and orthopedic surgeons around the world have included the Pilates method as part of their rehabilitative programs. For example, millions of people suffer from back pain—whether it's from poor posture, repetitive on-the-job action, or injury. The hallmark of the method is that each exercise addresses the spine. If done correctly, Pilates can alleviate most minor back pain.

The rumor was: Joseph could fix your body. Dance legends such as Martha Graham, Ruth St. Denis, and George Balanchine flocked to Joseph's studio to make his discipline part of their training. Rumor was that he rehabilitated, keeping in mind that physical therapy was not the sophisticated science

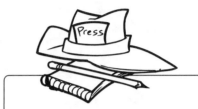

Pilates Scoop

There are two ways to work your body: a group Mat class or an individually instructed program. You can do both. Each Mat class was specifically designed to work your muscles in a logical sequence, and the apparatus are: the Universal Reformer, Cadillac, Wunda Chair, Electric Chair, the Spine Corrector, Ladder Barrel, the Magic Circle, and Ped-a-Pole.

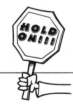

Pilates Precaution

If you have or had a back or knee injury, you should begin your reconditioning on the apparatus with the supervision of a teacher, preferably one who specializes in Pilates–based programs or a physical therapist who is trained in Pilates.

of today, an array of physical problems—aching backs to knees. And that's how his vision spread to you. Simply because his methods worked!

Many of those dancers were able to resume their professional dancing careers. Still, a handful of those dancers returned to New York to study with Joseph and Clara after retirement. In fact, these master teachers kept the "Movement" alive and vibrant. These devotees dedicated their lives to teaching and spreading the ideas of Joseph Pilates. Today, his exercises continue to thrive both for their recondition and fitness qualities mainly because his methods can be used by all walks of life!

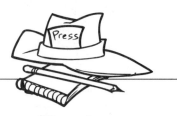

Pilates Scoop

Did Joseph Pilates invent the fountain of youth? He lived a long life, 87 years. His devoted wife, Clara, lived into her mid-80s as well. They both dedicated their lives to teaching the ideal fitness program in their New York studio.

Granny Got Her Groove Back

Like it or not, you're about to live a long life—on average, 80 years long, according to statistics—provided that you eat healthfully and exercise regularly. By exercising, you can protect against the development of high blood pressure, heart disease, cancer, depression, and osteoporosis. Exercise also can prevent disability and dependency, can combat stress, and can help you battle the bulge and sleepless nights.

There are hundreds of research studies to prove it—in fact, exercise can do more than just about anything known to medical science to ensure a fit, healthy, and happy life. Pilates can safeguard your body and mind and help you age gracefully.

Stay Stronger Longer

You're as young as you feel. However, staying young at heart requires a commitment from you. Whether you're 20 or 50, it's never too late to start an exercise program to grow old with.

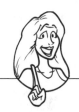

Pilates Lingo

Atrophy is a condition in which the muscles waste away to the point at which you can't engage in day-to-day activities. This doesn't happen because of old age, but because of an inactive, sedentary lifestyle. In fact, according to the American Sports College Medicine (ASCM), 250,000 deaths in the United States per year are attributed to physical inactivity.

Changes in your health and appearance are a normal part of aging, but you don't have to surrender. You can slow the aging process by eating the right foods and exercising. Wasted muscles happen because of lack of activity, not old age. Here's a fact: An active person will decrease $1/2$ percent physiologically per year, whereas, an inactive or unfit person will decrease 2 percent per year. Wasted muscles, a condition call *atrophy*, don't happen because of aging, but because we can't get off the couch.

Inactivity affects how you live from day to day; inactivity causes disease. If you continue to lose muscle fibers, the muscle will lose size and strength.

Stay stronger longer! You'll increase your odds of staying independent with the freedom to move and get about. With these exercises, you can slow but not stop the age-related loss in muscle size and tone, as well as prevent poor posture. With this discipline, you can build strong muscles and develop balance in your hips, legs, and ankles so that you can do activities that require quick movements. Imagine managing your own life into your 80s.

Battling Brittle Bones

Your bones are alive and kicking—in fact, your bones are continually remolding. You can have a lot to do with how the bone remolds itself by exercise and the way you eat. Your bones are made up of collagen and calcium. Collagen is a glue-like matter made up of vitamin C and water to make the structures of the body: skin, bones, teeth, blood vessels, cartilage, tendons, and ligaments—in short, connective tissues. Calcium is a mineral that's stored in the bones so that it can be used whenever it's needed for many of the vital body functions.

As the bones give up calcium, new bones are then molded. The body always needs calcium, so it recruits it from your bones even if the supply is low. This deficit, then, affects how the bones are remade. Eating a diet high in calcium is your first line of defense.

As you age, bone production slows; your bones lose the ability to reshape new bones. Over time, the bones lessen in density and become thin, brittle, and susceptible to fractures. This decay is caused by both the natural aging process and a disease called osteoporosis. This disease accelerates loss of bone tissue, making the bones brittle.

Signs of osteoporosis can be as subtle as rounded shoulders or as severe as a hump in the upper back. This hump, called a dowager's hump, affects 40 percent of the women who have osteoporosis.

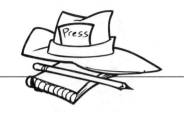

Pilates Scoop

Exercise is critically important in your golden years. A research study showed that men and women aged 90 and older increased their muscle strength more than 100 percent from lifting weights. Not only did they get stronger, but they were also able to walk better and take better care of themselves according to the book *Fitness After 50; It's Never Too Late to Start,* written by Walter H. Ettinger Jr., M.D., Brenda S. Mitchell, Ph.D., and Steven N. Blair, PED.

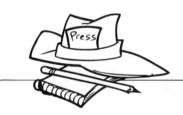

Pilates Scoop

According to the Kaiser Institute on Aging, the metabolic rate drops about 2 percent per decade. After age 35, you'll have an increase in body fat and a decrease in bone density at the rate of 1 percent per year. You'll suffer more postural changes and a loss of connective tissue.

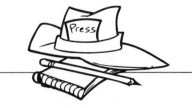

Pilates Scoop

Women have less bone mass to start with than men. During menopause, the ovaries stop producing estrogen, which protects against bone loss. After 50, bone loss in women starts to accelerate. Osteoporosis is the leading cause of bone fractures in the older population, causing an estimated 1.5 million fractures a year in the United States.

The good news is, the rate of bone loss can be slowed by regular resistance training. Yes—Pilates! The equipment utilizes springs to give you resistance while you use your body as resistance during the Mat workout. In other words, this discipline gives you the same results as a weight-training program does. In addition to exercise, make sure that you get good amounts of calcium, and, in women, use estrogen-replacement therapy after menopause. Study after study shows that walking and resistance training can slow the rate of bone loss, which helps prevent fractures and change in posture.

The best thing you can do now in your 20s, 30s, and 40s is to build your bones early in life. A diet high in calcium and plenty of Pilates can help.

Did Joseph Pilates invent the fountain of youth? His exercises kept him fit; he lived well into his 80s. Possibly you, too, can grow old with it. After all, growing old gracefully will soon be the in thing!

A Pea in a Pod

Pregnancy is kick-back and slack-off time—except when it comes to your body. After all, your body is about to change: more dimples, more stretch marks, more fat on the spots you've worked so hard to tone.

What you need at this time in your life more than anything else is lots of pampering: flowers, gifts, romantic dinners, and passionate kisses from the guy who put you in this temporary state of big-belly. Still, you can give yourself and your baby the best gift: good health.

Pilates provides the perfect combination. It prepares your body for pregnancy by keeping your abs and pelvic muscles strong, keeping them flexible and toned while carrying. It also helps you get your body back after delivery. Nine months of pregnancy is nothing compared to reviving your bod!

Is It for You?

Your body, your mind, and your soul all experience a series of ups and downs during pregnancy—more downs, perhaps, than ups. Some women glow from head to toe; others can't lift their head out of the toilet bowl. Swelling, constipation, backache, fatigue, bloating, varicose veins, and nausea are common woes. Can Pilates help? You bet.

Regular exercise during pregnancy helps to overcome some of the physiological and emotional changes—that is, if you're able to get out of bed. These exercises can reduce many of the annoying aches and pains of pregnancy, but is it for you?

You might be looking for an exercise program that's nonimpact and that tones your body. You've heard good things about Pilates: It strengthens the ab, tones the body, and doesn't put much stress on the body. All are true. So, you're thinking, "Great, I'll do these exercises while I'm pregnant."

Know this: It's not an exercise program that you should start in pregnancy. However, if you're shopping around several months prior to pregnancy, then Pilates is a good choice.

The exercises may seem like a good choice, but you're strengthening muscles that haven't been used before, especially your abdominal and back muscles, and you're creating extra stress by trying a method that is quite complex.

Taking charge of your health is empowering—it's good for you if you're planning ahead. If so, here's why these exercises can keep you healthy during and after your pregnancy:

➤ The exercises help develop strong abdominal muscles *before you get pregnant* and maintain them during pregnancy, two of the biggest gifts you can give yourself.

➤ Strong abs support a growing fetus.

➤ The exercises strengthen your back muscles, which can relieve lower-back pain from carrying the extra weight in your belly.

➤ The exercises keep the pelvic floor muscles in tone for delivery and help you to get them back after delivery.

➤ The movements are controlled—no jerky moves to put you at risk of overstretching your ligaments and joints.

➤ The exercises prepare you for breath work.

Pilates Precaution

One caveat: Pilates is a great maintenance program during your pregnancy only if you have been practicing Pilates prior to your pregnancy; it's not advised to start Pilates after you become pregnant. Consult with your medical doctor or care provider before exercising during pregnancy.

Listen to the Doctor's Orders

As with any exercise program, use common sense. If you're planning to get pregnant, then talk to your doctor. Pilates can help alleviate some of the discomforts of pregnancy if you take a few safety precautions. The do's and don'ts:

➤ Do ask your doctor for the current guidelines given by the American College of Obstetricians and Gynecologists (ACOG).

➤ Do modify all movements; the goal is "maintain" abdominal strength and pelvic floor muscles, increase circulation, and control your emotions with your controlled breaths.

➤ Don't overheat your body; exercise in an air–conditioned setting in the first trimester of pregnancy.

➤ Don't overstretch; you may find some of the exercises easier because the hormones that are flooding your body relax your ligaments and tendons. Resist the temptation to push yourself.

➤ Don't jerk your body into a move; use slow and controlled movements only.

➤ Do consider hiring a personal trainer to work you out on the apparatus especially as your belly gets bigger; it's easier than the Mat work.

➤ Do listen to your body.

In the Pursuit of Excellence

Winners don't distinguish themselves by physical strength alone; It's the combination of physical and mental stamina that makes a winner.

Enter Pilates! This ideal fitness trains the brain and body simultaneously and harmoniously. The exercises train the body holistically by integrating mental tuning, visualization, and breath control, while the muscles gain strength and length. By practicing the exercises, an athlete or fitness buff can achieve that edge, the fire in the belly radiating confidence. Pilates can help you maximize your athletic performance.

Sweat Isn't Enough

Today's athletes have enhanced their performances and have greater staying power; it's not uncommon to hear about the athletes competing well into their 30s and early 40s. To train holistically, you must train the brain and body simultaneously and harmoniously.

How you sleep, eat, and take care of your mind are equally as important as the physical training. Today's competitors have customized training programs that emphasize nutrition, stress management, and innovative and creative training methods that include mental preparation and physical performance strategies.

There is no mind/body separation. The mind tells the body what to do. The body, in return, does what it is told, whether you're aware of it or not. The exercises developed by Joseph Pilates are holistic because they integrate the mind and the body.

Every move starts in the brain. In a sense, Joseph Pilates trained as an elite athlete. Top competitive athletes, serious sports buffs, and anyone seeking a greater sense of well-being and deeper unity of body, mind, and spirit can benefit by adding his exercises and guiding principles to a training schedule. Here's why:

➤ You'll achieve a level of self-mastery by integrating the mind and the body.

➤ You'll develop the muscles more efficiently by cross-training.

➤ You'll reverse or prevent muscle imbalances, which can be caused by your specific sport. Developing the muscles uniformly is the foundation of every move developed by Joseph Pilates.

➤ You'll speed up recovery after training or a competition.

➤ You'll improve your concentration; it's this honed concentration that tells the body what to do.

➤ You'll develop breath control.

➤ You'll become more body-aware and disciplined.

➤ You'll improve your focus.

➤ You'll increase strength and flexibility in areas that were once weak.

➤ You'll better your "edge" by boosting your self-confidence.

➤ You can recondition your body.

➤ You can prevent injury by keeping your body flexible and evenly strong and balanced.

➤ You'll build core strength.

Training is divided into two categories: psychological and physical. The physical training is the grueling hours spent sweating it out. The psychological training, by contrast, is a combination of mental skills such as goal setting, relaxation techniques, breath control, concentration, and visualization. These techniques can be useful to anyone who wants to develop a deeper mind/body/spirit union, not just athletes.

Joseph Pilates said it best: "One of the major results of Contrology is gaining the mastery of your mind over the complete control of your body." Doing his ideal fitness better prepares you to achieve self-mastery for your sport!

With Pilates, you're accomplishing two goals: training the brain while strengthening the body, as well as improving your training and performance, no matter the sport.

Pilates Scoop

The exercises integrate the mind and body; it's a 90-year-old method that encourages physical and mental control as it strengthens the body and the mind simultaneously and harmoniously.

Strength and Length

Strength in a muscle that is lengthened is the goal of most athletes. Let's take a classical ballet dancer. In most cases, she is extremely flexible, but she often lacks the strength in some movements. In contrast, a weight lifter probably has strength yet lacks the flexibility to move in a full range of movements. To a ballerina, lifting weights is out of the question for fear that her muscles will bulk up and she'll become muscle-bound; the weight lifter fears putting on a tutu.

You can have both—strength and length. You won't compromise strength or flexibility. Each exercise strengthens and stretches the muscles to keep the muscle long, not shortened. In the end, length in a muscle means more strength. Why? Because you're developing more muscle fibers within the muscle itself. Therefore, you might even be stronger. Recent studies show that those who stretch after weight training can boost strength gains by as much as 20 percent! In other words, weight lifters don't have to don a tutu!

The research backing the benefits of flexibility is overwhelming. There's not a person who couldn't benefit from flexibility work. You'll increase your range of motion, reduce the muscle soreness associated with the post-work, and calm your nerves as well. Here's the payoff: You can lift more, your golf swing is more complete, your fast ball is even faster, and your running stride is a little longer.

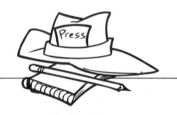

Pilates Scoop

You can develop more muscle fibers within the muscle itself, meaning that you might even get stronger by cross-training with Pilates. Recent studies show that those who stretch after weight training can boost strength gains by as much as 20 percent!

The Pilates exercises counterbalance hard-core training in two ways: by lengthening the muscle after it has been shortened or loaded to the max, and by cutting down on muscle soreness after your workout. There might be a link between lack of flexibility and post-work-induced muscle damage, according to the *American Journal of Sports Medicine*.

The more flexible you are, the less damage you'll have—although that's a hot topic for debate. Right now, there's not enough conclusive research to make that claim because injuries occur for a variety of reasons: lack of flexibility as well as muscle imbalances.

Risky Business

Think you're an in-shape athlete or sports buff? Look closely and take notes. Your muscles might have developed unevenly. Depending on the sport, some muscle groups are worked and loaded differently, while others are completely or partially ignored. Some overloading to the muscle groups can be caused by one-sided sports or by sports that completely don't strengthen certain muscle groups. Put another way, your muscles lack symmetry.

The Pilates exercises correct muscle imbalances, which is the foundation for every move developed by Joseph Pilates. Incorporating his work into your training schedule can put balance and symmetry back into your body.

Shattered Dreams

Staying injury-free should be your top priority as you refine your performance to attain elite status or your everyday fitness goals. Muscle imbalances, inflexibility, lack of self-mastery, plus a frazzled state of mind can all contribute to injury. Coping with an injury can set you back years, or maybe even shatter your dreams to compete.

No sport gives your body everything; you must *cross-train* to fill in the missing ingredients, whether it's to keep you sane or to train the muscles that are often neglected by your sport. Cross-training means practicing sports and activities other that your sport to build overall fitness. Overall fitness usually cannot be achieved with just one single sport.

A New You

Clearly, you can benefit from Joseph Pilates' life-long work no matter your age or fitness level. The most wonderful thing about practicing the Pilates exercises, besides all the mentioned benefits, is that you finish with a pleasant feeling, as if you just rejuvenated the mind and the body.

Take a look again at the benefits of the Pilates method:

➤ Strengthens your mind and muscles

➤ Enhances your breathing

➤ Increases your flexibility

➤ Redefines your body

➤ Redistributes your weight

➤ Stretches the body

➤ Eases the stressful aspects of your life

➤ Boosts your energy

➤ Shrinks your waistline

➤ Perks up your bottom

➤ Cures most back pain

➤ Heightens your sex life

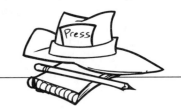

Pilates Scoop

There's not an athlete or sports buff alive who can't benefit from developing core strength, which is key to overall fitness. And most fitness experts agree that building a strong core is one of the best ways to prevent injury. Without core fitness, you'll get in shape to only a certain level, which means that you'll compete only so well.

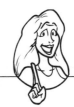

Pilates Lingo

Cross-training with the Pilates method can give you a break from your sport so that you can build overall fitness. Overall fitness usually cannot be achieved with just one single sport, so cross-training is a must to prevent injury, burnout, and overtraining, whether it's mental or physical.

➤ Builds your self-esteem and self-confidence

➤ Shrinks the dimple, an anticellulite solution

➤ Develops both strength and length in each muscle

➤ Strengthens your core

The Pilates movement is not just exercise. Instead, it is the way to lifelong fitness and mindful health; it promotes physical harmony within each of your muscles with an invigorating mind workout. Your goal is to use your mind to engage your body to perform these movements correctly. You will then experience a whole new you.

The Least You Need to Know

➤ Pilates, pronounced "puh-LAH-teez," engages you and leaves you refreshed and alert, with an enormous amount of self-confidence.

➤ Within every exercise, you'll work on gaining flexibility, strength, balance, and coordination.

➤ There are two ways to work your body: a group Mat class or an individually instructed program using the apparatus. You can do both.

➤ Pilates fulfills both psychological and physical training; it's a great way to cross-train for your own sport.

➤ Joseph Pilates's dream was for everyone to join the movement, from basic to advanced, from the injured to the super-fit, at any age and any level of ability.

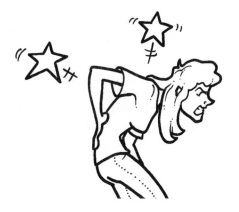

Chapter 2

Fix Your Frame

In This Chapter

➤ The message in your body

➤ Torso talk

➤ Getting a stronger, sexier back

➤ Getting rid of backaches and pains

➤ Striving for good posture

Call it grace, poise, self-confidence, or just plain sex appeal—some people have got it, and others don't. Do you want that demeanor that makes others stop and stare? Well, you no longer have to be an insider—"it" can be yours, effective immediately. Just follow the exercises developed by Joseph Pilates. They will lengthen your look and slim your midsection. The secret is a 90-year-old sequence of movements that works to gently elongate your back muscles, creating space between joints crunched by everyday life.

Message in Your Body

What message do you want to communicate about yourself when you enter a room? That you're strong? That you're confident? That you feel great about yourself? Let's say that you have a serious case of the slumps—your shoulders round forward. That message, then, may be that you're painfully shy? That you have no confidence? That you feel insecure about your height?

Consciously or not, we send a message about our mental, physical, and emotional state by the way we stand, sit, and move. Good posture projects good health, vitality, and confidence, while slouching can imply weakness, feebleness, and self-doubt.

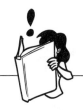

Pilates Primer

Studies show that good posture is more attractive than supermodel svelteness. In fact, a 125-pound woman can be perceived thinner than a 105-pound woman who is slumping, according to Don R. Osborn, an associate professor of psychology and sociology at Bellarmine College in Louisville, Kentucky. His research subjects consistently find women who stand up straight more attractive, regardless of their weight.

What's amazing is that this isn't a hot news flash. Most mothers, at some point, have instructed their children to sit up straight or pull their shoulders back. Current research suggests that people who have good posture not only are attractive to anyone looking at them, but they also look taller and thinner. That's right—no longer will you have to diet yourself to starvation to look slim; just fix your frame.

Torso Talk

You'll feel better about yourself—and look healthier, thinner, and sexier—by improving your posture. You can also protect yourself from a lifetime of annoying aches and pains.

You name it: muscles spasms in the lower back, compressed nerves that intermingle with the working muscles, chronic neck pain, recurrent headaches, decreased lung capacity. Good posture tames muscle strain and the aches and pains; helps you to move with ease, grace, and efficiency; and gives your lungs more working room by increasing breathing capacity.

So, how does your posture measure up? Are you slumping, rounding your shoulders as if you're protecting yourself? Perhaps you're craning your head forward to see the computer screen? Or maybe you're a slave to fashion and have to prance around in the hottest stilettos (which, by the way, cause you to arch your lower back). Whatever the case, you're committing a combination of postural offenses.

Ask a close friend or spouse to take a Polaroid picture of you. Don't pose. This shot needs to be as authentic as possible, so stand your usual way and strip down to your birthday suit, or your bathing suit, if you're too modest. Take several shots each of your front, side, and back views. After that, analyze your posture, starting from your head to your toes. Ask yourself these questions:

➤ Does my head hang forward?

➤ Are my shoulders rounded forward? Is one shoulder higher than the other? Or, are my shoulders tense, as if touching my ears?

➤ Does the upper part of my back hunch or round forward?

➤ Am I sticking out my chest, causing my shoulders to pull back? Are my shoulder blades sticking out?

➤ Do I have a potbelly—abdomen bulging forward—causing my lower back to arch?

➤ Am I locking my knees, causing me to arch the lower back? Or, do my knees roll inward?

➤ Are my ankles rolling inward as well, causing the arches in my feet to flatten and the knees to draw closer and closer.

➤ Are my feet splayed out, causing my knees to bow; in other words, am I bow-legged?

If you answered "yes" to any of these questions, then Pilates may help. But first, let's get acquainted with your spine.

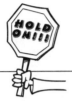

Pilates Precaution

Attention, women! Women tend to suffer from more aches and pains than men. For example, we're often slaves to fashion; we love high heels. As a result, we tend to suffer from lower-back pain. Wearing the hottest stilettos throws the pelvis into a forward tilt so that the lower back arches. Still, we tend to carry our children with the arm and hip on the same side of the body, which automatically raises the hip on one side and the shoulder as well. It's best to carry your baby in front, close to you, or to alternate your hips. Baby backpacks are great for newborns as well.

No More Pain in the Back

Poor posture stops here. The spine, sometimes called the vertebral column, consists of 24 interlocking bony blocks called vertebrae. Every vertebra stacks on top of the other, and these are supported by joints. The vertebrae provide back protection while the joints allow motion.

Then there are the body's shock absorbers, called discs. In between the vertebrae lie the circular, plump, jellylike discs that also allow movement. These discs cushion the vertebrae as you run, walk, and move. A finely balanced system of ligaments, cartilage, and muscles holds these vertebrae together and keeps the backbone from collapsing. And inside this structure is the spinal cord, a thick bundle of nerves. These

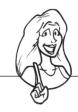

Pilates Lingo

Bone by bone means stacking your vertebra one at a time. This core concept is used in almost every exercise, so get used to peeling your spine up and down. Joseph Pilates used to say, "In coming up and going, roll your spine exactly like a wheel." Sometimes you'll read about "bone by bone," "vertebra by vertebra," "one vertebra at a time," or "peel your spine." It's all the same—move slowly and gradually.

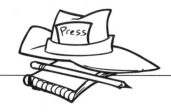

Pilates Scoop

Eighty-five percent of Americans have suffered from lower-back pain. Right now, eight million Americans have lower-back pain. In fact, back injuries are the most common on-the-job injury. And guess who's reaping the benefits? Drug companies; non-prescription pain relievers are a billion-dollar industry.

nerves thread between the spine's center to carry messages, including pain, throughout the body. With perfect precision, these groups work together. If the spine is lined up correctly—*bone by bone*—with balanced muscle groups, then back support can function without friction.

To feel the bone-by-bone sensation, find a tennis ball and try this experiment. Sit in a chair with your knees slightly wider than your shoulders. Place the tennis ball underneath your chin. Begin by dropping your chin to your chest to roll down your spine, one vertebra a time. After your hands reach the floor, peel your spine up bone by bone until your vertebrae stack up—the tennis ball will drop at that point. As you roll up, feel your vertebrae stack up to lengthen your spine. Get to know this feeling because it's a core concept in Pilates—you'll stack your spine in almost every exercise you'll do.

Strain, pain, and injury can strike any of these groups at any time. Ligaments and tendons, for example, can be strained or ripped. The muscles that support this system can suffer a pull. The joints can suffer wear and tear and become arthritic. The discs, a delicate, finely balanced structure between the bony blocks of your spine, can rupture just by lifting too heavy of an object. If a discs bulges, it may compress the nerves, which can be terribly painful.

Still, if the natural curves of the spine become exaggerated, then the bones press down incorrectly on one another, creating tension in some muscles while causing weakness in the others. Put another way, some muscles constantly contract as the opposing muscles lose the ability to contract and weaken.

A classic example is having too much arch in your back, which is commonly referred to as "sway" back—but that's not an accurate characteristic of this condition. The abdominal muscles eventually weaken while the back muscles strengthen. One result: a bulging belly. Your abs go on strike, so your back muscles must work that much harder to support your frame. Muscles become unbalanced, and you end up with an aching lower back. If your muscles can't support the body correctly, then perfect posture crumbles.

How Are Your Curves?

Healthy, pain-free backs are made. As we age, a lifetime of poor body mechanics, on-the-job repetitive actions, and too much hustle and bustle catches up. Some muscles weaken, causing others to tighten. Every back can benefit from these exercises because they restore strength, keep the spine flexible, and help maintain the natural curves of the neck, middle back, and lower back.

Take a look at your Polaroid pictures that you took earlier. Notice the natural curves in your spine. A healthy back has three natural curves and muscle groups that support the curves to help keep your back working fitly. An exaggeration of a curve, such as too much arch in the lower back, throws off the entire structure. Take a look at your curves:

➤ The cervical vertebrae are the most movable and make up the first seven vertebrae of your upper back, starting at the base of your neck (called C1 to C7).

➤ The middle of your back, called the thoracic region is the least movable and consists of 12 vertebrae (called T1 to T12).

➤ The lower back holds most of your body weight, and this is where the majority of back pain occurs. This is where you have your lumbar vertebrae, only five of them (called L1 to L5).

➤ Then there's the S1 to S5 vertebrae, the sacral vertebrae; these are fused into one bone. In most of the exercises, you'll be asked to anchor the sacrum to the Mat, which is the top, flat bone of the butt.

➤ Finally, there are four coccygeal vertebrae, which are also fused into one bone; this is your tailbone.

The spine really adds up to 26 active vertebrae. The sacrum is one bone, and the *coccygeal vertebrae* make up the other immobile bone. The other 24 bony blocks make up your curves.

Got a Slumper, Here!

Are a slumper? If so, you're particularly susceptible to annoying pangs of poor posture. Round your upper back forward, and the rib cage compresses downward to the hips. This decreases your breathing capacity, plus you've added an inch to your midriff, thus losing about 2 inches in height.

That slump causes your backbone to line up incorrectly, Common activities reinforce this exaggeration. Let's say that you spend most of your day typing on a computer, craning your head forward while your shoulders round. As the bones continuously stack up incorrectly, this causes friction, irritation, eventually pain, and wear and tear on the spine.

Compounding the problem is age. Did your grandmother shuffle around slumping her upper back? The *kyphosis posture* literally means an exaggerated curve in the thoracic spine, or upper back. That's one reason why your grandma lost a few inches as she aged. In addition to height shrinkage, slumping can have the following negative effects:

➤ Decreases your chest measurement.

➤ Causes your shoulders to round and narrow.

➤ Restricts your chest movement by pressing the rib cage down into your internal organs. Therefore, you won't be able to expand your lungs as much. The end result: shallow breathing, which reduces the oxygen flow to the body and brain, meaning less energy and vigor in your daily life.

➤ Creates a downward pressure, giving your heart, liver, and stomach less room to function.

➤ May eventually create cervical compression and neck pain.

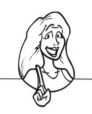

Pilates Lingo

Kyphosis posture means an exaggerated curve in the thoracic spine, your upper back.

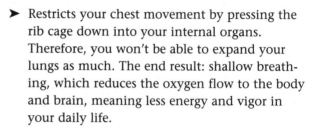

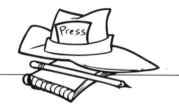

Pilates Scoop

Attention, men! If you can't live without your briefcase or laptop computer, then you could create a height imbalance between your shoulders and hips by lugging them around day after day on the same shoulder. Try thinning out the contents. If you still can't live without it, then alternate shoulders; otherwise, the muscle of the higher shoulder tighten and thicken while the other shoulder muscles weaken.

What's Up with Your Shoulders?

Got a hunch to go along with that slump? Chances are good that if you're walking around with a curve in your upper back, you're rounding your shoulders forward. So, what does that mean? The shoulder contains many bones that assist in moving the arms. Even the slightest exaggeration can throw off how the left and right shoulders work; a misalignment that's too forward or back causes the delicate balance of the spine to get out of whack.

Try this: Pretend you're Fonzi, from the popular sitcom *Happy Days*. Lift your thumbs as if you're a hitchhiker, but let your arms dangle by the side of your legs. Lift your thumbs up, pointing behind you to rotate your shoulders. Did you feel your chest open? How about a slight stretch across your chest? Your shoulder blades, the winged bones on your back, should have drawn slightly together.

Try this experiment again. This time, point the thumbs to your thighs to make your shoulders round forward. Here's the muscle imbalance: Your chest muscles shorten as the muscles in the back of the shoulder and between your shoulder blades lengthen, in which case you feel a constant tightness.

The point is, your shoulders should be in a neutral position. To do this, rotate your thumbs outward and gently bring your armpits to your hip. Now slightly draw the shoulder blades together to realign your shoulders. This way, the chest fully expands, giving your lungs more room to work. Put another way, you'll draw in no more shallow breaths; instead you'll breathe more deeply. Translation: more energy. Of course, it starts with fixing the exaggerated curve in your upper back.

Is Your Head Straight?

If you're slumping and rounding your shoulders, then check the position of your head. Does it hang forward? Lift your head as if a string was suspending it from the ceiling. The idea is to line your head directly over your shoulders to stay aligned with the body's center of gravity. This relationship between your head, neck, and back keeps the rest of your body in line: head, neck, upper back, lower back, hips, knees, ankles, and feet.

Been bowling lately? A bowling ball weighs as much as your head, 10 to 14 pounds. The muscles in your neck and upper back work around the clock just to keep the weight of a bowling ball in place. And that's why the tiniest move forward causes these muscles to work even harder, which initiates the downward spinal of poor posture.

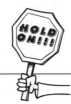

Pilates Precaution

Standing up straight as if a military drill sergeant only shortens the spine. Don't puff out your chest thinking that you're getting your spine straight.

This extra weight disrupts the body's center of gravity, which can slightly change the curve of the cervical spine and on down. Or maybe the slump caused you to hang your head forward. Whatever came first doesn't matter. This strain tightens the muscles in the back of the neck, which puts pressure on the joints and nerves that may result in chronic pain. A stiff neck, tingling or numbness in the arms and hands, and chronic tension headaches may be symptoms of poor posture. Look at the positions of your head, neck, and shoulders.

Too Much Arch in Your Back

Did you jerk up, jamming your shoulders back? So, now your chest sticks out along with the rib cage, quite possibly causing your lower back to arch? Don't worry; it's a common response to go the other way. However, you're setting off a different set of problems.

The *lordosis* posture often creates a dull, aching lower back as a result of too much curve or arch in the lumbar area. Even worse, you're weakening the abdominal

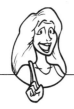

muscles. Look to see if your belly bulges out. In other words, belly muscles weaken as the back muscles overstretch. With that belly bulge, you're also getting these unfortunate side effects:

➤ Tight lower back muscles that can compress the sciatic nerve, which causes a dull ache or stabbing pain radiating from your back to the tip of your big toe

➤ Knees that are usually in the locked position to support the overworked back

➤ Feet that are turned in so that you're balancing the bulk of your body weight on the big toe and instep rather than the whole foot

➤ Tense, tight, often-lifted shoulders that weaken the upper back muscles

Are you locking your knees? Does your belly bulge? Or do you suffer from a dull, aching back? If so, pay special attention to your lower back because these are all signs that your bones are not stacking correctly. Try standing against a wall. Line your heels and shoulders up so that you feel them touching the wall. How big is the arch between the wall and your back? Is there a lot of extra room? Only the palm of one hand should fit between the wall and your back.

Putting Your Pelvis in Neutral

Come on, admit it! You probably haven't given your posture much thought. We get caught up in the daily grind, sitting for many hours in an incorrect position without realizing that we are reshaping our bones and muscles. Maybe we lock our knees while tilting our head to hold the phone in place as we talk and talk.

Take a moment and visualize all the parts of your body. Get a mental picture of the position of your feet, legs, hips, and buttocks. Don't forget your stomach and how you are holding those muscles. Visualize your spine and back. Ultimately, you want to create length in your body, especially in your spine. You're neither collapsing your shoulders too forward nor trying to stand up too straight, so your muscles and bones have a chance to *lengthen.*

Just by lengthening, you'll shrink your waistline, add a little height, add inches to your chest measurement, and provide more space for your working internal organs (such as the lungs), all while diminishing those annoying, nagging aches and pains that go hand in hand with poor posture.

To do this, you want the *pelvis in a neutral* position. You'll work a lot in a neutral pelvis position. Why? For three reasons: to lessen the arch in the lower back with hopes of reducing some of the pressure off your joints and nerves, to lengthen your spine, and to get you to use your abdominal muscles rather than your already over-worked back muscles.

Try this: Lie flat on your back and bend your knees. Feel the point or bony protrusions of your pelvis. These bony points are called the iliac crests. With the palm of your hand, rest your hand on this point so that it's flat. Even if you're in a neutral pelvis position, you might have a slight arch in your lower back. You don't want too much of an arch, however.

Lift your pubic bone to the ceiling to flatten the lower back to the floor; no light should shine through. You're tilting the pelvis into what's commonly referred to as a pelvic tilt. On the other hand, if you were to drop the tailbone into the floor, then you're creating an arch, and light does shine through. This is commonly called an anterior tilt. Experiment here. Tilt your pelvis back and forth (which feels great), and then return to a neutral position.

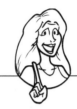

Pilates Lingo

You'll read the word **lengthen** a lot—it means to grow yourself tall. This length comes from the spine, as if you're pulled up from the top of your head by a string. Grow upward to achieve this length, bone by bone.

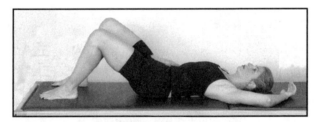

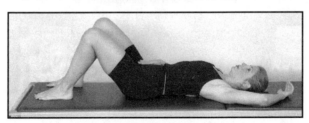

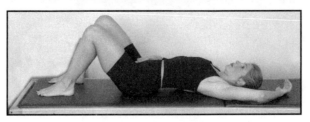

Top: In a pelvic tilt, notice how the fingertips lift higher than the palm of your hand. Center: Putting your pelvis in neutral. Notice how the hand flattens as it sits on the hip bone with your pelvis in neutral. Bottom: In an anterior tilt, notice how the palm of your hand lifts higher than your fingertips.

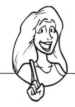

Pilates Lingo

To find a **neutral pelvis** on your body, feel the little bony protrusions toward the top of the pelvis, known as the iliac crests. With the heel of your hand, feel your pubic bone. Find the distance between those two points, and lay your hand flat.

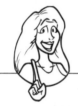

Pilates Lingo

Joseph Pilates coined the term **powerhouse**; it's your girdle of strength. The powerhouse sort of looks like a thick rubber band or corset that wraps around the middle part of your body; it expands from the bottom of your rib cage to the line across your hips and wraps around to your back. For most of us, it is the most neglected part of our bodies. You've seen it: the belly bulge.

Supplying Spine Support

However poor your posture is, it had help. The muscles that support your spine gave up at some point. Well, not exactly—they got that way through habitual patterns. Just about every exercise developed by Joseph Pilates addresses the spine in a three ways: to get you mentally working within your body so that you can break old habits; to strengthen and lengthen the muscles that support your spine evenly and uniformly; and to do every exercise in a biomechanically sound manner.

By rebalancing the muscles that support your spine, plus mentally focusing on fixing your frame, you can reverse the downward spiral of aches and pains over time. The bony blocks eventually line up correctly, which will eliminate friction, reducing inflammation and chronic pain.

Balanced muscles, therefore, make the difference between a healthy back and an aching one. Each fiber runs in a different direction to support spinal movement and create support for your trunk. So let's meet your muscles that help to support your spine:

➤ The trapezius muscle, or traps, runs from the base of the skull to the back part of the shoulders and then on down to the middle of the back to form a diamond shape. This muscle is often divided into the upper or lower trap. The upper trap lifts your head back and forth; this is also the muscle that tightens and tenses if you hang your head too far forward.

➤ The rhomboids are located in the center of your back. Try pressing your shoulder blades together; it's the rhomboids that protract them together.

➤ The biggest back muscle, the *latissimus dorsi*, wraps from the sacrum to the front ribs.

➤ The *serratus anterior* is located underneath your shoulders.

The Powerhouse

Don't let your stomach bulge; instead, use your *powerhouse!* The powerhouse links your abdominal muscles with your back muscles. To find your powerhouse, lie flat on your back. Place one hand on the bottom of your rib cage in front of your body and the other between your hips. Now inhale. As you exhale, notice how your belly button pulls back to the spine. That's your powerhouse pulling your navel to your spine.

Just about everything you do in life calls for your powerhouse. And that's why most of the exercises in this book work your powerhouse. As you train, your abs, hips, and lower back turn into a strong center of support so that you feel lifted whether you are just sitting or walking.

Work the powerhouse, and you'll flatten your belly, get rid of love handles, and firm up your entire backside. The muscles work to form a girdle of support for the middle of your body and spine. Get to know the layers of abdominal muscles—"abs," for short. Each fiber runs in a different direction to provide a strong support system for your trunk.

Try this: In a kneeling position, press your fingers below your belly and cough. Did you feel the muscle contract? That muscle, the *transversus abdominis,* stabilizes your spine because it's the deepest of the abdominal muscles; it wraps, sort of like a corset, from the bottom of your rib cage in the front to the ribs in your back and holds the visceral organs in place.

On top of the transversus is a set of criss-crossing muscles called the obliques. These muscles shape your waist and allow you to twist and bend sideways at the waist. If you point your fingers down toward the pelvis, you'll follow the pattern of the internal oblique muscles. The external oblique muscles, on the other hand, run up or the opposite way and lay on top of the internal obliques. Picture the letter *X*. Try bending and twisting at the waist to feel these muscles.

If you bend forward, you'll also feel the most superficial muscle, the *rectus abdominis.* It runs up and down the front of your body. Do a crunch, and you'll feel this muscle work.

By strengthening the core stabilizing muscles, you'll reap these rewards:

➤ Diminish upper- and lower-back pain

➤ Flatten your belly

➤ Shrink your waistline

➤ Lengthen your spine

➤ Fix your frame, for good!

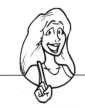

Pilates Lingo

Get to know your ***transversus abdominis;*** it will eliminate the belly bulge. You'll work all of your abdominal muscles evenly to create a firm flat center; however, the focus is on the deepest of abdominal muscles, the *transversus abdominis.*

Where's Your Body?

Clearly, posture matters. You should be aware of one thing, though: However poor your posture is, it might feel right to you. Start right now by thinking yourself taller. To do so, get in touch with how your body moves, and learn ways to control it. Quite frankly, that's how you'll get the most out of your workouts in the chapters to come, plus change your body.

Sure, every exercise works to correct posture, but it's not an overnight miracle. A certain amount of mental power will assist you. For example, you can prepare a mental checklist that looks similar to this one and practice standing tall:

➤ Stand with your feet hip-width apart to balance your weight evenly between your feet, knees, and hips. Keep your knees in a soft, unlocked position.

➤ Zip your abs by pulling your belly button to your spine. Remember the layers of abdominal muscles; it's the transversus abs that pull your belly in.

➤ Lift your rib cage slightly. Lengthen your rib cage away from your pelvis, for example, to reduce the pressure on your spine, which also shrinks your waistline. Still, this length helps to correct a rounded upper back, giving your lungs more space so that you can breathe more deeply. This also helps to realign your head over your shoulders.

➤ Unround your shoulders by gently pulling them up to your ears and rolling back and then press your armpits to your hips to draw your shoulders down, away from your ears.

➤ Relax your arms so that the palms of your hands face your thighs.

➤ Float your head up, as if a string was pulling it from the ceiling to lengthen your spine. You can gain as much as an inch in your height if you imagine this.

The plan is this: Align! Align! Align to train your body to feel what good posture is. Don't miss a day—align when you're sitting, standing, or driving. Tell your body what to do so that the body will follow; it's your matter, make it your mind. And, eventually it will feel like it's your own.

The Least You Need to Know

➤ Good posture projects good health, vitality, and confidence, while a slouch can imply weakness, feebleness, and self-doubt.

➤ These exercises lengthen your look and slim your waistline.

➤ The spine (the vertebral column) consists of 24 interlocking bony blocks that stack on top of each other.

➤ Your back has two functions: stability and mobility.

➤ Good posture relieves annoying aches and pains in the entire back—your waistline will shrink; your visceral organs will have more room to function better; and you'll breathe deeper.

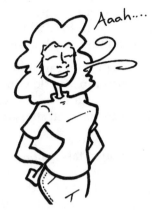

Aaah....

Chapter 3

Take Your Breath

In This Chapter

➤ Breathe like a baby

➤ Detoxify your body

➤ Become a better breather

➤ Breathe right

➤ Frost a window with your breath

It's a healthier way to wake up your body than, let's say, cappuccino. Breathing jump-starts your heart and gets your blood flowing. You can get your blood pumping to awaken every single cell in your body. This way, the body can carry away the waste and even win the battle of fatigue. In minutes, a clear and focused mental state takes over where sluggishness lingered.

Your breath is a life-enhancing basic. For example, you can't heal yourself without proper breathing. Everything from fatigue to stress-related health conditions can be alleviated by better breathing habits. By following the exercises in this book, you'll feel the mind-breath connection that Joseph Pilates purposefully planned to improve your state of mind and physical health. So, let's take a deep breath.

With Every Breath You Take

For thousands of years, "Yogis" have long claimed that the breath possesses the key to a healthier life and to clearer thinking. Westerners weren't so sure. Until recently, a flood of medical discoveries have found that good breathing techniques can enhance your overall health.

For example, you can use your breath to enhance your athletic performance; you can increase your stamina. Or, you can slow down your breath to tame tension, relieve anxiety, and improve other stress-related health conditions, such as heart disease.

If, for example, you slow down and deepen your breath, you can shift from a stress attack to a calmer mode; deep, slow, rhythmic breaths can also slow the heart rate and reduce a skyrocketing blood pressure. Slow, gentle breaths bring a calmer emotional state, which can be successful treatments for anxiety and stress-related heart disease.

Think about it. When you're anxious or angry, you often take gulped, hyperventilated breaths. This gasp of air reduces the amount of oxygen to your body, keeping you in a state of frenzy. Slow down your breathing, however, and you'll soon feel a "whoosh" of peacefulness penetrate your body. Use this same technique as a natural remedy for sleepless nights. Draw in as much air as possible, but this time exhale in a controlled manner as you count to eight. Set your mind free of the worries of the day that don't let you sleep at night.

If calmness is not what you're after, then you can use a percussive breath to increase your energy, to get the most out of life by way of enhancing your focus, concentration, and perhaps your memory. Coaches have used breathing techniques to help their athletes perform better, whether to calm their nerves or to pump them up for an athletic performance.

Could Joseph Pilates know this? You bet! You'll use your breath in a few different ways: to purify the body of the waste that makes you tired and to charge the body with oxygen to awaken all the cells in your body. And that's why he brilliantly choreographed each breath to every one of his moves.

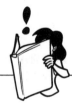

Pilates Primer

Words of Joseph Pilates: "Squeeze out the lungs as you would wring a wet towel dry. Soon the entire body is charged with fresh oxygen from toes to fingertips, just as the head of the steam in a boiler rushes to every radiator in the house."

In plain English, Joseph Pilates wants you to squeeze every ounce of air out of your lungs so you can inhale as much air as you can to charge your body with fresh oxygen—to give your body life! With every conscious breath, you'll feel healthier. Yes, good health is only a breath away.

Breathe Like a Baby

Pay attention to how you breathe. Are you breathing into your belly as if you don't have a care in the world? Or is your breathing restricted by your chest. If so, you're not alone. This could mean a few things. First, you've never been conscious of your breath. Second, you're emotionally blocked. Third, you never learned how to breathe correctly.

Have you ever watched the belly of a sleeping baby. Her little tummy rises and falls, effortlessly as if not a care in the world. That's one of the best examples of diaphragmatic breathing. You try it!

Unslump your spine and take a deep breath. Breathe in through your nose and let it travel down the back of your neck and then to each bone of the spine, lengthening as it goes and goes. Drag this breath out for a count of five. Try to make your belly rise. Could you do it? Not many can. And why? Because somewhere along the way you've forgotten how to breathe—and deprived yourself of the most precious gift. Oxygen.

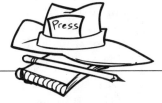

Pilates Scoop

The mind-breath connection was first discovered in India. When we're afraid, startled, or shocked, we hold our breath. The drama, then, stays with us long after the initial shock. By holding our breath, we lock the trauma in our bodies. Fear is said to be the root of many diseases. The Indian healing art of Ayurveda teaches you how to breathe properly, to unlock emotions that can eventually cure everything from depression to high blood pressure and stress-related diseases.

Discover Your Basic Breath

Life begins with your first breath, and it ends with your last. You'll inhale about 100 million breaths before your last one. Oxygen is the most basic need for life. The respiratory system includes the nose, the mouth, the windpipe, and the muscles that support the diaphragm and all parts of the lungs. Imagine what's happening in your body.

By definition, respiration is an event that exchanges oxygen and carbon dioxide between 60 trillion cells in your body. Breathing, however, is so much more:

➤ It carries nutrients to every part of the body. The cells within your body need oxygen to create energy and to carry out all their other duties.

➤ It increases your energy levels.

➤ It cleanses the wastes from your body. Toxic overload is one reason why you feel tired and sluggish.

➤ It calms you down.

➤ It connects you to your body.

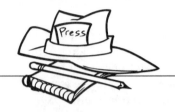

Pilates Scoop

You'll learn to breathe in a full, relaxed way that will increase oxygen levels for you, which can stimulate circulation and digestion. Deep breaths act like an internal massage for your organs, particularly the liver, abdominals, and heart, to make help them work more effectively.

Pilates Primer

Joseph says: "Lazy breathing converts the lungs, figuratively speaking, into a cemetery for the deposition of diseased, dying, and dead germs as well as supplying an ideal haven for the multiplication of other harmful germs."

Imagine two balloons. Picture them as they fill up with air; now let the air out. Your lungs basically work the same way. They fit snuggly in the vast space of your rib cage, in the body's chest cavity, filling up and deflating. As the lungs fill up and deflate, they act as an internal massage for your organs.

Between your ribs is a group of muscles, the internal and external intercostals. When you inhale, these muscles help to pull the rib cage out or expand your chest, while pulling the rib cage or chest wall in during the exhale.

Driving this action is your *diaphragm*; it's sandwiched between the bottom of the lungs and the top of the abdomen. This thin, dome-shaped muscle acts like a pump. As you inhale, it relaxes and moves downward, creating a vacuum, which sucks the air into the lungs. When you exhale, the diaphragm arches up into the chest to push all the air out of your lungs. Your ribs are going along for the ride, assisting anyway that they can.

You can feel this up-and-down action best by putting your hands on your belly. So, lie down. When you inhale through your nose, try to make your belly rise. Then slowly let all the air out of your lungs through your mouth while watching your belly shrink to its normal size. Think back to the sleeping baby. Its little tummy grows bigger as it inhales, filling air into the entire lungs; the little tummy then returns to its resting size. The baby doesn't fight the movement as her belly naturally rises and falls.

Let's say that your belly is not moving like a baby. Again, don't be surprised. For example, you may lose focus and let your mind wander. Or, perhaps you're used to breathing into your chest.

In that case, your diaphragm and intercostals aren't wholly operating, so breathing is restricted. And why? Because stress, tension, and suppressed negative emotions can constrict your breathing as if held hostage by your emotions. You're guarding! Truthfully, though, it's easy to forget how to breathe if you're not aware of your breath in the first place. We all take breathing for granted.

Is this a problem? You bet. As it stands, up to a third of the lungs consists of "dead space"—no fresh air gets into these areas. This stale air zaps your energy levels. Fill your lungs with deep breaths, and you can exchange that dead air for fresher air more frequently.

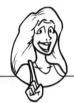

Pilates Lingo

Think of the **diaphragm** as a pump, sort of like an accordion that you push in and out to generate music. When you draw air in, the diaphragm relaxes and moves downward to create a vacuum. This vacuum draws the air into the lungs. To get rid of the air, the diaphragm contracts and rises up to push all air out of your lungs. To get more air, you need a good set of lungs; a strong, flexible diaphragm; in-shape and flexible rib muscles; and strong abdominal muscles.

Detoxify Your Body

Think of the lungs as organs of elimination that help purge toxins from the body. Cells in your body renew every minute; old ones die. Toxins accumulate through wear and tear on your cells. In addition, you inhale, eat, and touch all kinds of toxins; they, too, need purging. Toxins build up either internally or externally. Anything foreign to the body must be eliminated for optimal health.

Feeling sluggish? Unmotivated? Perhaps your zest for life has dwindled? These are all signs that your body may be suffering from a toxic overload, whether emotional or physical. You can really help yourself by breathing deeply. A trip to the bathroom is another form of elimination. Blowing your nose is yet another. The largest detoxifying organ is your skin—break a sweat, and you're definitely detoxifying.

Your goal, then, is to breathe deeply enough that all the cells in your body get enough oxygen. This can prevent toxic overload in the first place. But wait, let's back up. The body produces energy two different ways: aerobically and anaerobically.

Surely, you've heard of "aerobics"? By definition, *aerobic* metabolism means "with oxygen," while *anaerobic* means "without oxygen." Easy enough. Oxygen and lots of it, we know, enriches the body. Your cells thrive, and in return, you feel energized and alive, and that's what your body prefers. But what if there's not enough oxygen?

Two things happen. First, if the cells suffer from an oxygen-debt, there's a buildup of carbon dioxide. Second, for the cells to survive, they rely on the less efficient anaerobic method. This backup system is not the way to go for long periods of time. If you were to sprint away from an out-of-control car or lift a heavy couch up several flights of stairs, then an anaerobic state is the way to go. Not for long periods of time, however.

Besides being inefficient, anaerobic metabolism puts undue stress on the body; it produces a buildup of lactic acid and other waste by-products in the tissues. Muscles ache, and you feel fatigue. Have you ever pushed yourself to the point of exhaustion during a workout, chanting, "no pain, no gain?" How did you feel the next day, or the day after that? Like someone took a baseball bat to your body? One of the contributors to post-workout soreness is lactic acid. When your body rids of it, you feel better.

But let's say that you've lost some flexibility in your diaphragm and intercostal muscles, and both are not fully expanding. This happens if you're out of shape, when you age, when you feel stressed and hold tension, when you have tight abdominals, and when you're experiencing negative emotions.

You're breathing into your chest. As a result, the labored and shallow breaths are not delivering enough oxygen to your body. You've just initiated the downward cycle to bad health: Your body doesn't effectively purge lactic acid, carbon dioxide, and other waste byproducts of everyday living.

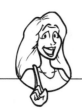

Pilates Scoop

Think of detoxifying as the body's way of getting rid of anything that it can't use. Drinking lots of water can help purge toxins from your body. In other words, anything that works to eliminate keeps you healthy. Making a trip to the bathroom, blowing your nose, or sweating after a good workout are some other forms of detoxifying.

Pilates Lingo

Aerobic means "with oxygen"; **anaerobic** means "without oxygen."

The good news is, you can reverse this downward spiral by avoiding as many toxins as you can—avoid cigarette smoke and air pollution, get plenty of exercise, drink lots of water, find an outlet for stress, and practice your breaths to strengthen and increase the flexibility of your diaphragm and chest muscles.

Work on Your Stamina

Need some flex in your diaphragm, or how about some stretch in your tight intercostals—both very healthy goals—to increase your lung capacity? What about building your stamina?

By definition, stamina, or endurance, is your capacity to perform longer without stopping to recuperate. Greater stamina, then, puts less stress on the body, and you might not suffer from a workout hangover—post-work soreness. You can achieve greater stamina with these exercises.

No, you don't have to lace up your running shoes. Deep, controlled breaths combined with non-aerobic exercises also increase your stamina. At first, some of exercises may be difficult, so you might need to rest before performing the next and the next. Use your breaths, however, to connect the movements so that each exercise flows into the next.

Eventually, your lung capacity increases because the two muscles driving breathing—the diaphragm and intercostals—strengthen. Both become more efficient and elastic. Now you've got muscle endurance. You'll be able to repeat the exercises without resting as much between moves. Not only will you replace flabby muscles for toned ones, but you'll also build stamina. This flow reduces the time that it will take you to exercise. Good news, right?

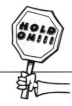

Pilates Precaution

Ninety years ago, Joseph Pilates instinctively predicted that overdoing exercise would do more harm than good. His exact words were, "This infraction creates muscle fatigue—poison."

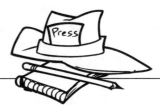

Pilates Scoop

Get high on Pilates! Why not? Studies suggest that deep breathing releases natural brain chemicals called endorphins. It's that feel good euphoria state that runners get after a good run. Guess what else releases endorphins? Laughter. Many students comment on how good they feel after a Mat class or a private session. Maybe they're suffering from a healthy case of endorphins. In any case, do it and laugh!

Become a Better Breather

"Even if you follow no other instructions, learn to breathe correctly," Joseph Pilates said. Yet, how do the exercises in this book help you to become a better breather?

➤ They help you become aware of your breath in the first place so that you take the first step toward being a better breather.

➤ They help you strengthen your muscles: the intercostal and diaphragm are both muscles that are imperative to optimal breathing.

➤ They help you purify the body of poisons, including lactic acid and carbon dioxide.

➤ They help you get in touch with your emotions. Deep breathing can bring repressed emotions to the surface.

➤ They help you to heal the body and the mind by learning how to breathe deeply.

➤ They help you relieve stress. When you're going through a stressful event, carbon dioxide levels rise as oxygen levels fall because you're breathing shallowly.

In these exercises, we breathe a little differently. We're still breathing deeply—deeply enough to deliver large amounts of oxygen to the body. But the emphasis is on the exhale; it must be forceful enough to get every ounce of breath out of your lungs— purify the body. Only then can you draw in a large amount of fresh air. You'll use the abdominal muscles to assist your breaths.

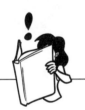

Pilates Primer

Joseph says, "Indefatigably and conscientiously practice breathing until the art of correct breathing becomes habitual, automatic, and subconscious, which accomplishment will result in the bloodstream receiving its full quota of oxygen and thus ward off undue fatigue."

Wrap your hands around your rib cage, with your thumbs on the back ribs and your fingers on the front. Inhale to open the rib cage, filling the ribs in your back with your breath. At first, this concept may be a little tricky for two reasons: You're not accustomed to breathing in your back—tight intercostal, diaphragm and back muscles have restricted your breathing. Your abdominal muscles also are weak.

Let's try breathing into your back: Lie down on your back with your knees bent and your feet flat on the floor. Put your hands around your ribs.

Inhale full enough to fill the lower lungs with enough air to expand the ribs in your back. Imagine an angel's wings expanding with each inhalation. Breathe along your spine. In other words, inhale through your nose, and let the air travel down your neck and spine, bone by bone, eventually to the ribs in your back. Even your shoulders flare out slightly.

Exhale through your mouth, relaxing the tongue and jaw as if you're frosting the window with your breath. Keep exhaling as you draw the belly button to your spine. Imagine your navel drawing up and under your rib cage.

When working with your breath, stay in a neutral pelvis; it's the abdominal and respiratory muscles that should work. Don't despair if you can't breathe into your back. This concept takes practice and some time to develop that kind of mental and muscle control. Your deep abdominal muscles, for example, have probably been neglected for a while; it's their strength that contributes to guiding your breath.

Practice breathing into your back so that you can get this feeling before you start the exercises. Inhale for five counts, and then exhale for five more.

Still, your breath protects you from injury. When you exhale forcibly, the deep abdominal muscles, the transversus and obliques, tighten around the spine to protect it, like a corset. If you're bulging your abs, then your spine is unprotected. Picture your abdominals as a corset around your spine, getting tighter and tighter.

The Rules: Breathe Right!

Breathe right, and soon you'll reap all of its benefits. Breathe wrong, and it might take some time before you notice your body changing. There are definite no-no's. Never hold your breath. Breathe in through your nose; exhale through your mouth. As with all rules, there's always an exception. However, most of the exercises follow these instructions:

➤ Inhale on the point of effort.

➤ Exhale to a relaxing position.

➤ Exhale to squeeze the body tight or in a closed body position, pressing every ounce of air out of your lungs to protect your back.

➤ Exhale to flatten your belly as much as possible, with no belly bulging.

➤ Inhale as you straighten up.

➤ Inhale to initiate each twist.

➤ Breathe for the duration of the movement to reduce stress and strain.

Pilates Primer

Joseph Pilates developed the breathometer, which was a small device that looks like a pinwheel connected to a straw. With the breathometer, he got his clients to breathe, which is essential to developing their potential lung capacity. If they could make the pinwheel spin, then they could actually feel the power of their exhalation.

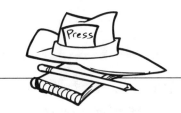

Pilates Scoop

As you blow all the air out of your body, pull your abs up under your ribs. If your belly bulges—like a loaf of bread— you're not protecting the spine. Think of your deep abs as a corset that gets tighter and tighter as you exhale.

➤ Don't hold your breath.

➤ Try pausing with your breath to let your insides expand.

➤ Breathe in through the nose, and exhale through the mouth as the jaw and tongue relax.

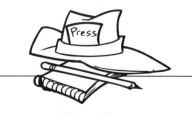

Pilates Scoop

Think of the inhalation as the in-spiration for your movement; this breath takes you through the point of effort.

Pilates Scoop

One liter of oxygen burns five calories.

Avoid Running On Empty

Obviously, you're breathing enough air to get by; otherwise … well, you know. But are you getting enough fresh oxygen to reach your full potential? Now, that's a different story. The fact is, if you're not breathing deep enough, then the body can't do its job. You know, the stale air hangs around in the bottom of your lungs, poisoning the body.

As you age, the problem worsens. You can lose flexibility in your chest and lungs. Why? Poor posture! Now, you're starting to see the brilliance of Joseph Pilate's lifelong work. If you don't work to correct poor alignment, then breathing is restricted whether you're young or old.

Let It Flow

Joseph Pilates warned his students not to hold their breath while working out. Besides creating an oxygen debt, it stresses the body. In other words, you're wasting precious energy on muscles that don't need to be involved in the movement. A relaxed muscle tone makes more energy available for the move itself.

Vow to Get More Air

Short on air? If you've been breathing into your chest, then you're not getting enough air. Let's try to break the habit. From this day on, make a vow to get more air. Remember, without the help of your abs, your diaphragm will not get to pump away. Your diaphragm is responsible for 75 percent of the air you get.

Chest expansion can't deliver enough air, mainly because the middle and upper chest interferes with air flow. That puts the thoracic breather at an oxygen debt. You're working harder to breathe, which puts extra stress on the entire system. The lungs work that much harder, as does your heart.

Again, look at your posture. Maybe you're rounding your upper back. If that's the case, then work toward fixing your frame. Perhaps you're feeling emotionally blocked? Then examine your lifestyle. Are you a type A personality? Is your life stressful? Do you suppress your feelings? Your joys? Your sadness? Years of tension can cause you to breathe into your chest. Enhancing your breathing capacity may help. You can also visit a breathing specialist, someone who specializes in emotional healing or bioenergenics, or see an Ayurvedic practitioner.

You're striving for freedom, emotional as well as physical. Get rid of the tension that holds you back from breathing fully and the good health that you deserve.

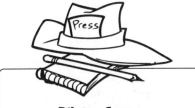

Pilates Scoop

Stand up and yawn. That's right, a yawn is one kind of breathing technique. It is usually a result of a buildup of carbon dioxide in the blood. If this waste reaches a certain level, then the yawn reflex is set off, releasing the stale air that sits deep in your lungs.

Trust Your Nose

Attention mouth-breathers: Stop it! You're supposed to breathe through your nose; it's much healthier. Here's why. The nose heats the air and gets it ready for your body. And then there are the thousands of microscopic hairs inside your nose, called cilia. The waving motion of these hairs filters the air before you take it in the body. In other words, pollution, dirt, or anything else that's not supposed to enter the body is rejected by the *cilia*.

Your nose, then, is the first line of defense in the detoxification process. Nothing gets past your nose. On a similar note, exhale through your mouth. Don't purse your lips together as if kissing someone. Instead, relax the tongue, lips, jaw, and face.

Tune Up Your Breath

The Pilates method teaches you breath awareness first. However, you may need to seek the help of a loved one or hire a breathing coach to help monitor your breathing patterns. Definitely pay close attention to your moods and how your body holds stress. For example, you may hold your breath on every minor crisis in your life and don't know it.

Start a breathing diary. Think about your breaths at this very moment. Have you ever been in a situation that caused you to feel tightness in your chest? Write it down. How do you feel after an argument? For example, do you hyperventilate and gulp for air? In most cases, unpleasant events trigger breathing irregularities. If left unchecked, then the cumulative effects can cause tight intercostal muscles or inflexible diaphragm. The good news is, both are muscles—you can lengthen and strengthen them. The bottom breath is, are you getting your quota? Why not, then?

Monitor your breath while doing the exercises in this book. Look for instances in which you stick your tongue out and hold your breath, as you may have a natural tendency to do as you learn new movements.

Use your breath to help with a move. Exhale to release muscle tension, and relax the not-working muscles so that you have more energy for the working ones. Stay calm, and breathe. Always remember the words of Joseph: "Even if you follow no other instructions, learn to breathe correctly!"

The Least You Need to Know

➤ Good breathing helps your performance, reduces stress, increases your stamina, and detoxifies the body.

➤ Good breathing may help defy many of today's most costly stress-related diseases—heart disease, anxiety, asthma.

➤ Full, deep breaths get rid of toxic wastes that make you tired.

➤ By definition, respiration is an event that exchanges oxygen and carbon dioxide between 60 trillion cells in your body.

➤ One liter of oxygen burns five calories.

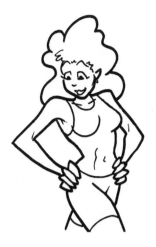

Chapter 4

(Re)Discover the Perfect Body

In This Chapter

➤ The art of training

➤ How the Pilates method complements other fitness programs

➤ Metabolism makeover

➤ Pilates training tips

One day you put on your favorite pair of blue jeans and think, "Whoa. What's going on here?" So you strip down to nothing and check yourself out in a full-length mirror. Hmmm. Your narrow hips don't look so narrow. You have a little extra bumper power around your back end. And your legs don't look as slender as they used to.

"That's it," you say with finality. You decide that you need an exercise program that will keep you motivated. No more erratic workouts, and you vow to curb your insatiable appetite. You need a fitness tune-up, Pilates-style.

Spring to Life

Have you fitness flat-lined? Not only is your mind bored, but your body as well; it's resisting change. The Pilates exercise program helps you trim and tone your body, but not overnight. You'll have to make a commitment to working out, staying faithful to yourself. The ideal fitness won't change your body if you work out only once a month; you have to work at it! Making a wish list will help: "I wish I had buff buns." "I wish I didn't have to sweat during the workout." "I wish my arms didn't jiggle as much." Wishing won't change your body; commitment to the "ideal" fitness will.

The exercises in this book build up your body, not break it. Joseph Pilates said, "The workout leaves you as if you're springing out of the shower, not dead."

Yes, you'll be physically challenged, but not sore. Even if you feel a little frustrated, please don't give up!

The Art of Training

Even if you're an Olympic contender, don't be surprised if you can't roll your spine off the Mat. At first glance, these movements seem easy; yet, they are very complex. As Joseph Pilates put it, "Most professional athletes couldn't do their exercises properly when they started." That's why you have to concentrate while doing these exercises—it's the will of the mind that tells the body to do what you want it to do.

Pilates Primer

According to Joseph, "Ideally, our muscles should obey our will. Reasonably, our will should not be dominated by the reflex actions of our muscles."

So, get ready to engage your mind to move your body. It's easy to do, if you remember the following guiding principles:

➤ Concentration

➤ Control

➤ Centering

➤ Flow

➤ Precision

➤ Breathing

All principles are interrelated with each move you make, giving your mind and body a makeover.

Concentrate on Your Moves

Sure, Pilates tightens and tones your body, but it won't happen without the help of your brain. It's this fusion between the mind and the body that drives you to move. Introducing the first principle: concentration.

Concentrate on each move: the position of your head, the point in your toes, the arch or flatness in your back, the bend in your knees, and the rhythm of your breath. If you can *visualize* the exercises correctly, then you will do them correctly.

Control is Crucial

If you don't move with control, you can injure yourself. Make sure that carelessness doesn't carry over

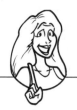

Pilates Lingo

Today, many athletes use **visualization** to strengthen their inner power so that they can achieve the results they want. Train the brain, and your body will physically respond.

from everyday life. Clear your head before you work out. Quick, jerky moves don't deliver results any faster; they only lead to injury as the wrong muscles work. Be in control of your body, not at its mercy.

Discover Your Center

Have you ever studied yourself? Not just looked in the mirror to find a few flaws, but actually watched your body as it moved? Go on, check yourself out. Don't focus on the ripples; rather watch your midsection. All motion starts here, in your center, a.k.a. the powerhouse. Your center muscles support the spine, the internal organs, and your posture. By building a strong body foundation, you'll trim your waist, flatten your belly, improve your posture, and move with grace and ease.

Every time you work, the focus will be on building a strong center. The work will appear in many different forms, but you'll always be working it. Motion flows outward from your center; hence, the fourth principle is flowing movement.

Find Your Flow

Make the exercises flow. Movement should always initiate from your powerhouse with control and continuity. Never rush through any direction—no jerks! And don't throw your body into the movement if you don't have the strength. You can modify all moves so that you can progress safely to the next level without injury. Haphazard, jerky, and stiff movements are all no-nos.

Move with Precision

Picture the Olympic games. Think about the ice skater making three full turns in midair, or the high diver flipping through the air. These movements, no doubt, are complex, but these athletes make them look so easy, as if we could do them.

Of course, we know that these moves are executed with sheer precision and mind control. What's the difference between a perfect 10 and a very good 8? No doubt, both routines are great but it's the performer who flips with grace, ease, and perfect timing that earns the 10.

The Pilates moves call for the same type of precision. First, learn the steps to each exercise along with the breathing patterns. Don't forget about the guiding principles: Concentrate on your body, do each move with control, initiate these moves from your center, establish a flow between steps, and follow through with precision. In other words, fine-tune your moves; precision is the icing on the cake.

Precision transcends into your ordinary life. It affects how you walk into a room, how you sit, and how you carry yourself through life. Think through these principles every day so that you can go through life a little more graceful and mentally balanced.

Build Your Breath

Finally, each step coordinates with your breath. Controlled breathing purifies the body, builds stamina, and reduces stress to the body when carrying out the exercises. Even better, you'll find that your thoughts are not as clouded. Pure, rich blood floods your organs, including the brain, with every breath you take. Deep breathing sends your body buzzing. And don't forget about the basic rules of breathing:

➤ Inhalation is the inspiration for your movement.

➤ Breathe into your back, to keep growing from within.

➤ Squeeze the corset a little tighter to get all the air out to make a pinwheel spin.

➤ Never hold your breath.

Pilates Primer

Joseph says, "As a heavy rainstorm freshens the water of a sluggish or stagnant stream and whips it into immediate action, so Contrology exercises purify the blood in the bloodstream and whip it into action with the result that the organs of the body, including the important sweat glands, receive the benefit of clean, fresh blood carried to them by the rejuvenated bloodstream."

Metabolism Makeover

Honor those muscles, find peace with the imperfections, and engage your mind to give your body the makeover that it deserves. How? By increasing your muscle mass so that your body burns more fat. That's what these exercises do—they increase your lean-muscle ratio, just like pumping iron does. However, instead of lifting weights, you'll lift, twist, stabilize, and control your body to get weight-training results without Herculean bulk.

Train Yourself to a Better Body

Maybe you didn't know this, but you've got the power to influence how your body burns calories—that is, increase your lean muscle mass and reduce overall body fat. It's true, buff bodies burn more calories during the day than flabby bodies.

Your *metabolism* is how the body uses fats, carbohydrates, and proteins in the form of energy; it's how you burn calories. Whether you're doing absolutely nothing, running from soccer game to soccer game, or just breathing, your body uses calories.

The concept is easy. Heat the body, and you'll burn more calories; cool down your body, and you burn fewer calories. Guess what? Muscle needs more energy to function than fat; it requires more calories during the day, even if you're lounging on the sofa.

The good news is that this discipline super-challenges your muscles. You can build lean muscle and reduce your overall fat; in doing so, you'll burn more calories during the day to shape up your body. Why not wake up a sluggish metabolism? Crawl out of bed and start exercising. During a 24-hour period, the metabolic cycle operates much like everything else in life; it speeds up during the day and slows down at night.

You might feel sluggish when you wake up, but so does your metabolism. By noon, it's picking up speed; by dinnertime, it's peaking; and by bedtime, it's falling. So forgo that cup of java, and work out with Joe!

Eat Yourself Healthy

You can also give your metabolism a makeover by eating. Hold on—don't sprint for the refrigerator just yet. It's true, though. Eating raises your metabolism; this process is called thermogenesis. The body requires energy just to digest the food and absorb the nutrients from the foods you eat.

Metabolism peaks at dinnertime. It slowly progresses as the day continues, so let's keep your metabolism peaking all day, especially at the low points during its cycle, by grazing on six small meals a day. Even though this caloric burn is small in comparison to exercise, it adds up. But you can get double the caloric burn by exercising and eating a snack in the morning, when your metabolism is still sleepy.

As another plus, you won't go hungry by healthy snacking. It's a better way to control your weight, especially if you have an erratic work schedule that forces you to skip meals. If you skip meals, you might have a tendency to play make-up-a-meal by eating everything in sight. You can end up eating a lot more calories this way than your body can use.

Don't forget to factor in healthful eating tricks. Eat mindfully. Rather than stuff fast food down your throat, have a smoothie that combines two to three fruits to get five or more servings of energy-giving foods. You can also squeeze your own juice. For example, add a few carrots and Granny Smith apples, and you have a healthy pick-me-up. Now you're ready for Pilates.

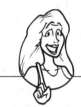

Pilates Lingo

The **metabolism** is how the body burns calories. You can be doing absolutely nothing, and your body will still burn calories. You can alter your metabolic rate by increasing your lean muscle mass and reducing your overall fat.

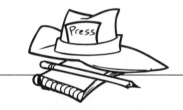

Pilates Scoop

Create a Picasso plate. That is, every time you eat, try to consume as many colors as possible, such as leafy greens, multicolor peppers, and a wide range of hues from berries. The more colors, the more disease-fighting protection you'll take in.

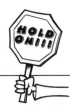

Pilates Precaution

This fitness can be a wonderful way to get your body in shape and can work as a preventive program for many health ailments. However, it is imperative that you consult your physician, especially if you are pregnant, before starting any exercise program. Please get a checkup: blood work and a pressure reading, a cholesterol count, a stress test, and a flexibility test, just to name a few.

Train Yourself Right— in *Six* Weeks

Ask yourself this: What do you want from this fitness program? Chances are, you started other fitness programs and dropped out because your goals or expectations were not met. Or, maybe you want to add a new dimension to your existing program? In any case, write down a list of wishes. Do you want a completely new look? Do you want to drop a few pounds? To get slim and sexy? To tighten and tone just a few jiggly areas? To be able to reach your toes? To fit into your favorite pair of Levis? To rid the annoying aches and pains?

Let's make a plan of body-attack. Decide on a time to exercise. Morning workouts tend to be easier to squeeze into a busy schedule. By getting it over first thing, you won't have to battle all the annoying interruptions of the day. What's more, that feel-good feeling stays with you long into the day. Yet, deciding on the perfect time will clearly be a choice based on your personal best hours, whether you're a night or a morning person. Whatever the time, make a commitment, and don't miss your workout.

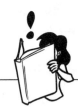

Pilates Primer

Joseph says, "If you will faithfully perform your Controlology exercises regularly only four times a week for just three months, you will find your body development approaching the ideal, accompanied by renewed mental vigor and spiritual enhancement. Controlology is designed to give you suppleness, natural grace, and skill that will be unmistakably reflected in the way you walk, in the way you play, and in the way you work. You will develop muscular power with corresponding endurance, ability to perform arduous duties, to play strenuous games, to walk, run, or travel for long distances without undue body fatigue or mental strain."

Decide how long you want to exercise, keeping in mind your goals. If slimming down your body is your wish, then exercise at least 45 minutes to an hour. If toning is your goal, then you should exercise 45 minutes. Be realistic. If you've never exercised before, then take it slow, perhaps 30 minutes, eventually you can progress to an hour workout. In addition, set a six-week review to witness the transformation, no matter how slight.

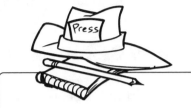

Away with Aerobics? No Way!

Maybe you're a die-hard aerobics queen. You love to spin your heart out, or you enjoy the climb on the Stairmaster. However, you're intrigued by the lure of the "ideal" fitness regimen. Do you have to give up your current exercise program? No way! Just squeeze in the occasional Pilates session.

The majority of my students already train in some other forms of fitness. Some spin, while others take aerobics; some still lift weights. Besides the muscle challenge, they want variety in their fitness. That's a great idea, because that's how you make a lifetime commitment—by mixing things up.

> **Pilates Scoop**
>
> Is once a week enough? Absolutely! Many of us do other forms of fitness and can squeeze in the "ideal" fitness once a week. The strength, flexibility, coordination, and balance work, plus breathing techniques will come in handy in life and in your own favorite fitness. You can also reap posture benefits. Obviously, the more you do, the more you'll get out of it—but some is better than nothing!

The Not-So-New Fitness

The question is, how will you ever know if your body is changing? Easy. Take some Polaroid pictures of your posture as suggested in Chapter 2, "Fix Your Frame," or find some old photos of yourself. You'll be much more committed to achieving your goals if you actually see some improvement. And pictures never lie.

To refresh your memory, you'll want to strip down to your birthday suit, or your bathing suit, if you're a little modest. Ask a loved one to take the shots. Snap an entire roll, focusing on the front, side, and, of course, your rear end. Don't be shy. Even if you don't like your back end, you have to have a starting place. You'll definitely find your body, flaws and all.

In addition, get hold of a tape measure, and measure the circumference of your arms, waist, derriere, and legs. Jot down these numbers. Now jump up and down and take note of what wiggles. Your goal is to tighten anything that moves. Stay away from the scale.

After 6 weeks, you'll retest with hopes of attaining the first steps toward your fitness goals. For example, let's pretend that your goal is to squeeze into a pair of pants, a pair that you haven't worn in a while.

Don't deviate from your pledge to the ideal fitness. To reap the benefits, exercise four times a week, for at least 45 minutes each day, and complete six weeks before looking at those pictures. "Practice faithfully; let nothing sway you," Joseph Pilates used to say.

Body Beautiful, but Not in a Day!

You won't learn everything overnight. Notice that the exercises are divided per chapter. This was done so that you can safely progress to the complete workout. The introductory Mat exercises span a six-week period, but you can advance when you feel comfortable. You do want to push yourself—after all, it's a workout.

Your goal is to learn all the introductory moves and breathing patterns, keeping in mind the six guiding principles at all times. After six weeks, reevaluate your progress. At that point, add a few of the advanced moves to your routine to keep the mind and muscle challenged. Here's a warning: The best ways to learn the Mat exercises are through repetition and by layering as the weeks go on. Don't progress too quickly; otherwise, you might get frustrated if you can't do the movement. Let's divide the weeks with respect to how you'll learn the exercises:

➤ The Beginner work, **Weeks 1 and 2:** You'll focus on 10 moves, and each one can be modified. Let's face it: Learning the moves along with the breathing patterns will be enough of an introduction. Try to complete at least eight to ten workouts with these moves before advancing to the next level.

➤ The Beginner–Intermediate work, **Weeks 3 and 4:** You'll learn five new moves, plus a couple of training tips to fine-tune your workout. Try to complete at least eight workouts with all the exercises up to this point.

➤ The Intermediate work, **Weeks 5 and 6:** You'll learn seven new moves, plus training tips. These exercises complete the introductory work.

Pilates Primer

Joseph says: "Correctly executed and mastered to the point of subconscious reaction, these exercises will reflect grace and balance in your routine activities."

Your ultimate goal is to pay attention to each move and to execute each motion with every ounce of control and precision, coordinating each breath every time.

Joseph Pilates didn't just teach his method; he embodied healthy living. In his book, he writes about getting plenty of sunshine and fresh air; not overeating, because it's dangerous to your health; getting a good night's sleep each night; and using a good, stiff brush to clean out the pores and remove dead skin because the pores of the skin must breathe. These were visionary claims 90 years ago, and now the science is here to prove him right. Don't you think he's a man worth following?

The Least You Need to Know

➤ The six guiding principles of Pilates are concentration, control, centering, flow, precision, and breathing.

➤ Your muscles should obey your will.

➤ You can make over your metabolism by increasing your lean muscle mass and reducing your overall fat.

➤ Do the "ideal" fitness four times a week to make over your body.

➤ You don't have to give up your current fitness program—just make time for a Mat or a private session.

Part 2
Show Me the Mat

There's a reason why Pilates is so fashionable. It works! In Part 2, you'll learn the core concepts, terminology, and Mat exercises. The exercises taught in this section are the same moves taught by Joseph Pilates. I'll introduce you to the exercises in the correct sequence so that you can develop your body with muscle symmetry.

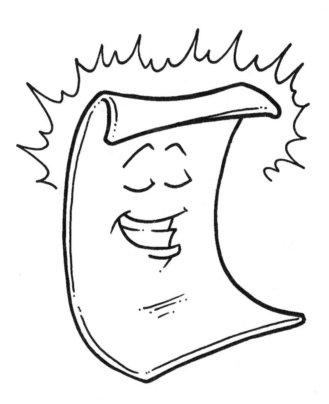

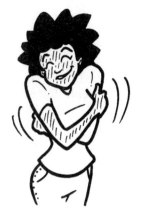

Chapter 5

Befriend Your Body

> **In this Chapter**
>
> ➤ Work from within
>
> ➤ Your body takes the path of least resistance
>
> ➤ Learn the concepts
>
> ➤ Mini-exercises to train your body

Go ahead, crunch your heart out; squat until you drop, and curl until you're jiggle-free. No matter how hard you pump, looking your best comes from within. There is a certain "it" that brands a body beautiful—the way you hold yourself in any position.

Joseph Pilates understood the secret to attaining poise and grace. And now fitness experts agree. You need to work the body to achieve total balance and synergy between all your muscles. Don't despair. You can still tighten and tone the most eye-catching parts. However, the smaller, often forgotten muscles need a little attention, too—they perfect the way you look and move.

It's never too late to make weak muscles strong. The exercises in this book reveal muscles that you may never even know you possess. But before you start, you'll need to know how to stabilize your body against movement. Enter pre-Pilates! You'll practice several mini-exercises that teach you how to get in proper position for the actual exercises that will soon follow.

So, consider this a warm-up; it's a way for you to get in touch with the new muscles that will be working and to get you to know your body a little better. In a sense, you'll befriend your body!

Body Wisdom

The goal is to know your body. Imagine that your bones are covered in layers of muscles. Let's divide these layers into two groups: *stabilizing* and *movement* muscles. In other words, the inner deep or stabilizing muscles hold the body in place, while the much larger superficial muscles move it. The essence of Joseph Pilates's work is to develop the muscles evenly so that the muscles hidden below, behind, and between the more well-known muscles develop as well. In a sense, you're working from within because many of these muscles support your frame. The *transversus abdominal*, the deepest abdominis muscle, provides a band of support around your midsection, for example.

Movement muscles, on the other hand, are often superficial. You can feel them move your body. The abdominal muscle *rectus femoris*, for example, is probably the one you're most familiar with, especially if you've done a crunch or two. This ab muscle bends the body forward and lies close to the surface. This muscle is often strong, probably from overtraining.

You can be fit but still be weak if you neglect these not-so-well-known groups of muscles. If they get weak and give into gravity, then the whole body tends to sag, or the working muscles get stronger while the weak muscles get weaker. This imbalance can create poor posture and eventually lead to a variety of aches and pain, initiating a vicious cycle.

Let's say that these muscles are weak from poor recruitment, meaning that the nerve impulses that control all muscles can't get through the muscle. Poor recruitment happens for two reasons: First, the muscles haven't been used enough. Second, pain occurs.

Let's say that you're suffering from an aching lower-back pain. Most back pain, we know, is caused by poor posture. More than likely, you didn't work the muscles symmetrically in the first place. In any event, you've got pain, and you don't think it's a smart idea to work out with this pain.

Alleviating pain is the right thing to do, always! Yet, question why you have pain. Ask yourself, "Is my aching back a result of me never working it or not working the muscles evenly?" This mental review is the first step. After you rule out anything serious, then you can formulate a plan. If your back aches because of lack of muscle recruitment, then you need to devise a plan that works the muscles of the spine and abdominals evenly; otherwise, you'll continue to create imbalances as nerve impulses dwindle in certain sets

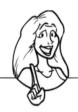

Pilates Lingo

Stabilizing muscles are often deep muscles hidden between, under, and behind some of the more common muscles, while movement muscles tend to be superficial in nature. An example of deep abdominals includes the **transversus abdominis;** the **rectus abdominal,** on the other hand, is a movement muscle.

of muscle groups. Put simply, the muscles waste away! You know the saying, "Use it, or lose it." It's never so true as for your muscles.

Training with Symmetry: Muscle Imbalances

Our bodies will always take the path of least resistance, even if we're engaged in the most mundane task. Our bodies cheat, no matter what the task, because it's part of our subconscious.

Pretend that you're a tad high-strung, with clenched, rounded shoulders that remain somewhere near your ears. This, we know, causes the chest muscles to weaken while the back muscles overstretch. However, your body doesn't suspect a thing; it prefers to function on a day-to-day basis this way, even during exercise. Not only will you have to recondition your body, but you'll have to do the same for your mind.

The brain must be aware of bad body habits; only then can you alter your appearance. It's a two-step process, or else you're reinforcing bad body habits that show up later in life in the form of a twinge, a spasm, or an ache. The body is a closed system, meaning that if one part is out of alignment, then the entire structure is altered. Misalignment has serious repercussions: Posture problems can affect internal organs' functions. So, while clenched shoulders aren't pretty, your breathing also may be compromised in the process, and that will dull your vivacious vitality.

A symmetrically developed body is a beautiful one. Many bodies, however, lack symmetry. We're programmed to go for the burn. Many forms of fitness, then, contribute to or promote imbalances by further weakening the stabilizing muscles. After all, we're working harder and doing faster movements to get that burn, instead of doing slow and controlled moves that develop muscle symmetry.

This imbalance leaves us aching, our joints overstressed, and our bodies vulnerable to injury. We've got tight and strong superficial muscles, while our very important stabilizers weaken as time goes on. Muscles work in groups, never alone, to move your body. One group will contract while the opposing group lengthens to move you. Some muscles overwork; others underwork. Muscles can become too tight or too loose, depending on how you use the body. We know that this imbalance upsets your structure, and it's only a matter of time before you ache. To correct the imbalance, you must do four things:

➤ Stretch the tight muscles, often overworked muscles, usually the superficial ones.

➤ Strengthen the weak muscles, often deep stabilizing muscles including postural muscles.

➤ Correct any alignment problems.

➤ Develop core strength and stability.

That's the essence of Joseph Pilates's work—you'll flex and stretch within every exercise to put symmetry back into your body. You don't have to figure out how, because (thanks to Joseph) the exercises are perfectly arranged to work the muscles evenly. Just to give you an example of his brilliance, you'll "center" your body during every exercise by focusing on the abdominal muscles as a group to provide a stable base of support. Developing core strength is the very first step to attaining symmetry in your body.

For example, if you have too much arch in your lower back, then your tendency will be to perform exercises with too much arch. In other words, you haven't corrected the problem; you've only strengthened the muscle imbalances. If you don't correct the problem first, by centering, for example, then you won't restore balance to the midsection, which could protect your lower back from injury in the long run.

You must have a certain amount of body wisdom to recondition the muscles, realign the body correctly, and change it for good. Sadly, we're not always aware of bad habits. So, here's the first step: Pay attention to your body. For example, pay attention to how it moves all day. Find habitual patterns, such as cradling the phone receiver in the same ear as you talk, carrying your child with the same arm, or engaging in a sport that uses the same muscles. Remember this: you'll have to tell your body to move differently. Otherwise, it will not change.

Pilates Primer

Joseph says, "Contrology develops the body uniformly, corrects wrong posture, restores physical vitality, invigorates the mind, and elevates the spirit."

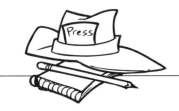

Pilates Scoop

The three main body parts—neck, shoulders, and hips—are balanced over each other. Your center of gravity is behind your belly button. You'll see it again, but start to think: neck, shoulders, and hips.

Your Cheating Body

Remember the first time you tried to ride a bike without training wheels? You might have the scars to prove it! When was the last time you pedaled away? If you were to hop on a bike today, your knees would probably be spared the scrapes. Your muscles would pedal without you thinking about it; it's called muscle memory. You don't have to think about walking, after all. Your muscles do what they know best as a result of repeated moves for many hours. Put another way, your body automatically responds.

New tasks, however, require a certain amount of concentration. The mind moves your body. Movements don't initiate in the bones, but deep inside an area of the brain called the *cerebral cortex*. This happens unconsciously in a matter of moments. You see the movement, and then the nervous system determines the best way to move your muscles.

Therefore, reeducating the body is not always an easy task. Many of the exercises that you will do require concentration; it's a mind challenge even for a skilled athlete. A marathon runner is often in great shape, with thighs lean and strong. His leg muscles can run for 26 miles, but if he were to perform a Roll-Up, then he might not be able to do it because he lacks core strength and flexibility.

It doesn't matter whether you're an athlete, a first-timer or a client with poor posture—you'll need to concentrate, control, and focus on good positioning. If you don't set up the body correctly, then the body cheats. Why would it work any harder than it has to?

Our muscles do the same. Stronger muscles, therefore, overcompensate for the weaker ones because it requires less effort. The marathon runner, for example, unconsciously depends on the strength of his strong thighs to get his body to do the Roll-Up. His muscles are asked to do something new, a move that he doesn't have the strength for. So, the muscles cheat, and his body follows along.

Eventually, your muscles will respond. Before long, you'll subconsciously know how to position the body. That way, you can build strength in areas that were once weak to have that "it" look. Remember, Pilates initiates in the brain!

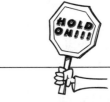

Checking Out Your Form

Say it again: Neck! Shoulders! Hips! Run through this mental checklist before every exercise. Proper body position is vitally important to the integrity of the exercises. If you don't fire the muscles correctly, then the moves are less effective. You also might not get the body you want.

While conditioning the body, you'll train the brain to work the same way every time. Start with the neck, torso, pelvis, each limb, and your feet. This firing pattern starts at your head and ends with your big toe.

Pilates Precaution

When do you call it quits? Whenever you're tired, can't focus, or don't feel comfortable with the movement. If you can't keep good alignment while doing the exercise, then the movements are ineffective. You don't have to complete the recommended reps—one perfectly executed move beats any number of sloppy ones.

Initiation: Learning the Concepts

You can learn all 500 exercises, but that doesn't mean that you know this discipline. However, if you master the concepts, you'll reap these rewards:

➤ You'll continue to grow, not get bored.

➤ You'll strengthen and stretch all your muscles.

➤ You'll correct muscular imbalances.

➤ You'll fix your frame.

➤ You'll get the body you want (within reason, of course).

➤ You'll take what you've learned in Pilates and apply it to other areas of your life or your fitness life.

If you memorize just the exercises, you'll get just that—exercises. In this case, you might get bored or unmotivated to work out if you can't continue to challenge yourself. This is not true only for Pilates, but also for any sport.

If you learn the philosophy, you can do any move anywhere, and take what you've learned in Pilates and apply it to other areas of your life, especially other forms of fitness. You may want to train with a private instructor or attend Mat class, let's say, in Australia. In this case, the delivery may differ from coast to coast, depending on the instructor, but the core concepts are universal. Feel these core concepts in your body, and let them enhance your life, whether it's improving athletic performance or slimming your body.

You're about to learn a series of mini-exercises that teach core concepts. Each mini-exercise will help you to get the most out of your workouts to come. This approach is gradual; it's a way to develop a solid foundation.

You can advance as you feel fit. Use your imagination and creativity to get the most out of exercises now or 10 years from now. You never know—you might be engaging in a Pilates class in Italy in the near future.

Learning the Lingo: Pre-Pilates

Pilates has a language all of its own. Phrases such as "roll your spine off the Mat," "bone by bone," "scoop, scoop, scoop," and "navel to your spine" conjure up all kinds of images. This is good because imagery helps. In other words, if you read "stack your vertebrae," then mentally picture your spine stacking one vertebra on top of the other. You'll read these phrases throughout the book. Have fun, and do exactly as it reads.

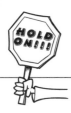

Pilates Precaution

Stabilizing the body before it moves is extremely important because it protects the body from injury and works the muscles more efficiently.

To do these exercises safely and correctly, you must learn how to stabilize your body against movement. This is an extremely important point: If you don't learn to stabilize the body before moving, it will move incorrectly or will move into the joint, which is typically weaker than your muscles.

So, let's start by learning how to stabilize the main areas of the body with a few mini-exercises. You will always work evenly in the trunk!

Transforming Your Transverse: Scoop

Think navel to spine! Imagine scooping your belly button in to make the distance between your stomach and your lower back smaller and smaller, as if the abdominal wall is right up against the spine.

Ever squeezed into a pair of jeans, lying on a bed and sucking in your stomach just to zip them up? It's the same contraction. The lower abdominals pull the belly button to the spine so that you can zip up your pants. However, don't just suck in your gut; it's a less violent way to pull the belly button in and up into the rib cage. You might feel the spine lengthen and your back anchoring to the floor; these are good signs. You try it: Take a deep breath. Slowly exhale as much air out of your belly so that the belly button pulls in as you zip up, up, and up!

By now, you're familiar with the superficial layers of the abdominal muscles: the rippled six-pack look of the rectus abdominis and the obliques. But the muscle that you really want to get to know is the *transversus abdominis,* or the transverse (in this book the two terms are interchangeable). This is your deepest abdominal muscle, and you'll use it in every exercise to develop core strength and to get what everyone desires—a flat, beautiful midriff.

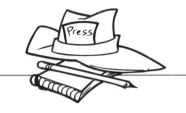

Pilates Scoop

The transverse abdominal muscle is vitally important to every exercise because you'll use it to develop core strength, slim your center, and protect your back. To get in touch with the deepest abdominal muscle, put your hands around your waist and cough. Notice how the abs get a little smaller with each cough; it's the transverse that pulls your belly button to your spine.

With a controlled, full exhale, you must get the abs closer and closer to the spine. Look for belly bulges on the exhale. That means that you're not scooping enough to get the navel to the spine. In this case, you're not working the right muscles, but building a belly bulge! By pulling your navel to your spine, you're doing the following:

➤ Lengthening your spine

➤ Stabilizing your center

➤ Strengthening the often neglected powerhouse by putting symmetry back into your core

➤ Getting rid of the belly bulge

➤ Developing core strength

Transform your transverse with the "Pregnant Cat":

1. Get on your hands and knees, as if you're a pregnant cat.

2. Inhale and drop your litter of kittens to the floor—hence, bulging your belly.

3. As you slowly exhale, pull your belly button in and up to your spine, without arching the spine. Stay in neutral spine so that the belly exhales in and up.

4. Repeat the exercise a few times until you can feel the transverse work.

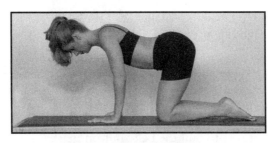

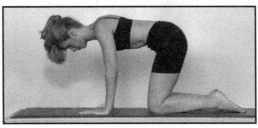

Spine to Mat

"Spine to Mat" works together with "navel to spine." Remember, in and up! Whenever you read "spine to Mat" or "anchor your spine," imagine that your torso weighs 50 pounds; it's heavy and is anchored to the floor. There's no light between your back and the Mat. Do this now: Lie on the floor. Try to feel every vertebra in your backbone and the back of your shoulders.

Pilates Primer

Joseph Pilates called the center "a girdle of strength." All movements initiate from your center.

This "heavy" feeling protects your back from injury, plus develops powerhouse strength. To get this feeling, lie on the floor on your back. Lift your legs in the air, with your toes reaching to the ceiling. You should feel every vertebra sink into the floor as the spine lengthens and anchors itself to the Mat. That's the feeling you're going for, as if making an imprint of your spine in the sand. Now, lower your legs slightly to challenge the back and abdominal muscles. Did your back arch? If so, you're probably not engaging your abs, or you might not have the strength yet.

Peel Your Spine off the Mat

If your spine is on the Mat, then you have to find a safe way to come up. "Peel your spine off the Mat" curls the vertebrae one at a time off the Mat, bone by bone. Think of peeling your spine up and down as a wheel turns.

Stacking your vertebrae, bone by bone, works the powerhouse, increases the spine's flexibility, and protects you from injury as you roll up and down. You must always protect your back—no jerky movements. From a "spine to Mat" position, peel up, feeling each vertebra as in bone by bone, called *spinal articulation*.

"Imprint" your spine while peeling up and down, as if you're making a duplicate copy in the sand.

Peel your spine off the Mat with these steps:

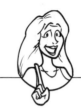

Pilates Lingo

Peeling your spine off the Mat, or **spinal articulation,** protects the back as you roll up and down, increases the flexibility of the spine, and works the powerhouse.

1. Lie on your back with your knees bent and your feet flat on the Mat. The pelvis is in neutral position as you press your sacrum into the Mat.

2. With your arms at your sides, focus on releasing the tension in your neck and shoulders. Let all the muscles along the spine relax as you sink into the Mat, making a duplicate copy in the sand.

3. Inhale through your nose to feel the rib cage widen into your back.

4. As you exhale, sink your sacrum into the Mat, starting to lift the pubic bone toward the ceiling. Feel each vertebra as it imprints into the sand.

5. Inhale down bone by bone. Repeat three times.

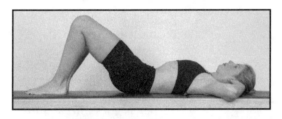

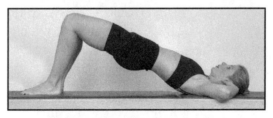

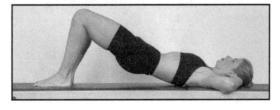

Propelling Your Pelvis: Pelvic Clock Work

As you imprint, imagine that your pelvis is wearing the face of a clock: The pubic bone is 6:00, while the base of your breastbone is 12:00; the left hip is 3:00, and the right hip is 9:00. The spine starts between your ears and ends between your legs. So, you'll do a series of pelvic clocks to bring awareness to your spine, massage your sacrum, and get you in touch with your powerhouse, which is housed in the pelvic region. To do this, you'll move the lumbar spine from flexion to extension.

In extension, the tailbone moves to the ceiling to lengthen the spine. Notice that the pelvis moves to a posterior tilt. If you've done a crunch, then you're very familiar with this position. If you move the tailbone to the floor, then the pelvis moves into an anterior tilt and shortens the spine; that's flexion. And neutral pelvis maintains the natural arch in your lower back—not too arched or too flat. You'll learn to drive this movement from the powerhouse, not the glutes and hamstrings, which may be ingrained in your head after years of doing crunches.

You'll use this core concept over and over again. For example, as you roll up from the Mat, you flex the body forward to activate the abdominals to bring you up—hence, forward flexion. As you come down, curl the pelvis by lifting the pubic bone to the ceiling (hence 6:00), continue curling to the 12:00 position located on your breastbone. Notice how the belly "scoops" to form a letter "C"—that's called a 6-12 pelvis curl; it's much safer to initiate the movement, plus you are forced to use your powerhouse instead of your back muscles—or, worse plopping down. It's this scoop that will transform your transverse!

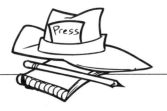

Pilates Scoop

Rocking the clock is a way to massage your sacrum, warm up the pelvis, and get you in touch with the powerhouse, which is housed in the pelvic region.

Refer to the figures in Chapter 2, "Fix Your Frame," to practice your pelvic clocks:

1. As you inhale, the tailbone will naturally sink in the direction of the 12–6 curl; it's okay if the pelvis goes into an anterior tilt.

2. Exhale and slowly lift the pubic bone to the ceiling in the direction of a 6–12 curl. Repeat three times, and then return to a neutral pelvis position.

After that, you can lift the bone of the pelvis to the ceiling or 3:00, while sinking the other bone into the Mat, at 9:00. Then reverse the times, 9–3; rock side to side to relax the powerhouse. Then rock the clock by moving from each point, starting with 12:00.

Chin to Your Chest

The head is in line with the spine the whole time! The spine starts between your ears and, because it's heavy, "chin to your chest" is the safest position for your head, neck, and back. It works in line with gravity to hold your head in a safe position.

Try this: Anchor the back of your head to the Mat. Then place a tennis ball between your chin and your chest. Or, if you don't have a tennis ball, then take hold of your ears and lift your head out of the neck without dropping the chin to the chest. Do you feel how that position creates length in the back of your neck?

This length stretches your neck muscles in the back, while strengthening the neck muscles in front and safely honoring the head, neck, and back alignment.

Most students at first can't hold their heads up, whether it's because of tight muscles, lack of strength, or pent-up tension. Don't strain to hold your head up; instead, put one hand behind your head for support, or lower your head to the Mat when it gets tired. As you develop neck strength, you'll hold "chin on chest" for longer periods of time. Let's try two easy mini-exercises.

Practice chin to chest:

1. Get into position, with your pelvis in neutral. Anchor the base of your skull into the Mat, creating length in the back of your neck. If you're arching your neck, put a towel behind the base of your head to prevent you from arching your neck.

2. Lower and lift the chin, with very subtle nods. Repeat five times.

3. Then clasp your hands behind your head and take a few normal breaths.

4. Inhale and lift your chin to the chest.

5. As you exhale, sink the breastbone into the Mat, and relax the neck and jaw muscles—you should be able to talk in this position.

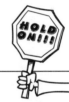

Pilates Precaution

Don't jerk your chin to your chest. Create length in the back of your neck, and then lift the chin to your chest. The spine starts in your ears, so always work with the head in line with the spine; most exercises will initiate with chin to chest alignment.

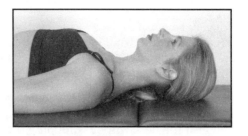

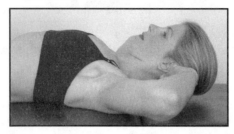

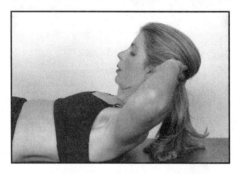

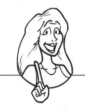

Pilates Lingo

The ***serratus anterior*** is a broad, thin muscle that covers the lateral rib cage and that connects to your shoulder blades. It holds your shoulder blades in place, which helps to stabilize your shoulders.

Pits to Your Hips

Don't "hunch your shoulders," Joseph Pilates would say. That's not always easy, though. For one, that's where many of us hold our tension, in the upper back. Second, the back muscles that support the spine are often weak. And finally, these are some of the most overworked muscles in the body.

Give yourself a hug! Feel the winged bones that stick out of your back? These bones are your shoulder blades, or scapula. These bones, along with a few muscle groups, keep the spine erect and stabilize the shoulder girdle. Try this: Bring your shoulder blades together. Do you feel your chest open as well?

Before any movement, we stabilize the shoulder blades. In fact, these exercises strengthen the muscles that stabilize the scapula: the muscles between your shoulder blades, the rhomboids; the muscles that depress the shoulder blades, the trapezius; and the muscle that holds it in place, the *serratus anterior.*

If you press your shoulders back and then down, you'll feel the connection between these muscles. Scapula stabilization is vitally important to your posture and to protecting the joints in the shoulder girdle. Remember how the body lines up: neck, shoulders, and hips! In other words, stabilize the neck, shoulders, and hips to align the body.

Stress throws off this connection. And because we're not always aware of pent-up tension, the problem compounds. After all, can you tell? Shoulders glued to the ears, or one shoulder higher than the other are true signs that you need to relax. So relax and strive for Pits to your Hips—shoulders down always!

Practice this:

Feel the scapula draw down the back in this exercise:

1. Go into a sitting position.
2. Clasp your hands behind your head, and draw your shoulders up to your ears.
3. Draw your shoulder blades down your back, and feel the muscles that are preparing you for movement—remember, Pits to your Hips!

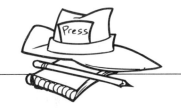

Pilates Scoop

We overuse the muscles in the neck and shoulders. These muscles overtense and cannot rest or be released, so they remain active, in a constant state of contraction. Over a period of time, the muscle can't reach its normal length, and the movement becomes resisted—hence the "Quasimodo look."

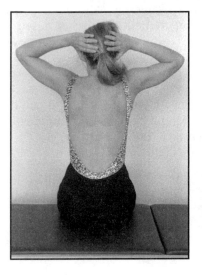
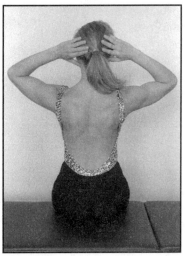

Pinch, Pinch, Pinch Your Butt Cheeks

Put a thousand-dollar bill between your butt cheeks and squeeze—at least, imagine it. Buzz words such as *squeeze*, *pinch*, and *tighten* should conjure up images of a tight bottom! But why? Of course, to work all the right areas: the butt cheeks, the upper back of the inner thighs, and the ever-so-vital pelvic floor muscles that keep your internal organs and muscles from dropping out of your body—imagine a hammock wrapping from the base of your pubic bone to the anus. Perhaps most importantly, hip stabilization works in conjunction with the belly muscles to develop core strength and stability.

Think about sipping a thick milk shake through a straw. As you suck harder and harder to bring up the thick milk, your face cheeks dip in. The same thing is happening here, except that you're pinching your butt cheeks. This contraction tightens and tones all the right places, so if you can't do this on your own, then put a small ball between your thighs and squeeze it to tighten all those muscles. Keep it there until you can activate these muscles on your own.

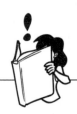

Pilates Primer

You learn to stabilize the trunk before any movement takes place. So, the focus is on three centers of control: Trunk stabilization—the deep abdominals (transversus, and internal and external obliques); scapula stabilization—midback muscles (lower trapezius, serratus anterior, and rhomboids); and hip stabilization—pull up through the inner thighs and pelvic floor muscles.

Pinch, Lift, and Grow Tall

Try this: Face a mirror. Sit up tall, and imagine that a string attached to the ceiling is lifting your head so that you grow taller, bone by bone. Keep lifting so that the rib cage separates from the hips, yet don't splay the ribs. This length must come from your spine as the head floats up, lifting every bone. Now, pinch your butt cheeks so that you grow even taller. That's pinch, lift, and grow tall!

Joseph Pilates would say, "Sit up out of your hips." This position is a neutral pelvis, meaning no tilting the pelvis. You can really feel this connection if you sit directly on top of your *sitz* bones, or butt bones. Try this: Sit on your bottom, with your legs straight out in front of you, but don't lock your knees. Grab the flesh from underneath your bottom, and pull it away from the bones. Sit directly on top of those bones. Now scoop your belly and pinch your butt cheeks—pinch, lift, and grow tall!

If you can't keep your pelvis in neutral spine, then put a little pad underneath your bottom. Tight hamstrings and overdeveloped hip flexors can interfere with this connection.

Pinch, lift, and grow even taller with this mini-exercise:

1. To grow even taller, reach underneath and feel your butt bones.

2. Lift the flesh so that you can sit directly on top of your sitz bones.

3. Now pinch, lift, and grow tall.

   If you can't sit up out of your hips, put a small pad underneath your bottom. This picture is an example of not being able to pinch, lift, and grow.

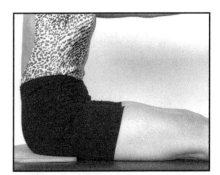 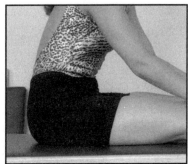

Just for Feet

Put work in your feet—take it out of your seat! In other words, don't point like a ballerina. Curling your toes over can throw your legs out of line with the rest of your body—or, worse, can cause muscle cramps in your feet. Lengthen, instead, from the top of the big bone in your foot, and then let the toes fall into a soft point.

If you're asked to flex the foot, then lengthen the heel away from your face as the toes reach to the body. You'll feel a stretch in the back of your calves. But be careful—overflexing can cause your leg muscles to cramp, too.

Before You Go!

You can do these mini-exercises any time. Trunk and midback stabilization, along with learning to lift through the back of the thighs and pinching your butt cheeks, are vitally important core concepts, not only for your safety, but also for the development of your muscles. You're striving for symmetry.

Keep in mind these core concepts that you learned will stay with you no matter how you choose to train, with the Mat or with the equipment. You've got to learn to stabilize the body for movement.

With that, extend it! Always think long from the powerhouse. You can reach a little farther, which is not only true for Pilates, but as a fact of life—extend, extend, and extend!

The Least You Need to Know

➤ The three main body parts—neck, shoulders, and hips—are balanced over each other.

➤ A neutral pelvis balances the head, neck, and shoulders to line up the body.

➤ Legs and arms move from the core, your powerhouse.

➤ Stabilize the body against movement.

➤ If you memorize just the exercises, then you'll get bored. If you learn the concepts, then you'll grow—and that goes for any fitness that you may choose.

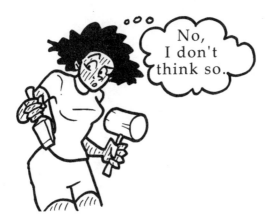

Chapter 6

Sculpt Yourself into Shape

In This Chapter

➤ Body awareness is everything in Pilates

➤ The mind influences the body, and vice versa

➤ Ten top moves

➤ Understanding your scoop

Chances are, you've lifted hundreds of sets of dumbbells and kicked your body into kick-butt shape. You might have been the first to fasten your bottom to a very uncomfortable bike seat to Spin, and you might have found inner peace through yoga. Indeed, you might have sweated with the best of them. You're the boss of your body, and you're ready for the next challenge.

The movement featured in this chapter is the most effective way to introduce your body to the Mat workout. You'll use your body as resistance to lengthen your look, strengthen your muscles, and chisel your core. Along the way, you'll inspire yourself to do more, learn more, and be more as you beam with confidence—even in this first stage—as you conquer more.

A Perfect 10

You'll cover a lot of ground in this chapter, so keep in mind a few things. These exercises are balanced and arranged to work your muscles symmetrically, thanks to Joseph Pilates. Do the exercises in order. In the first two weeks, do these beginner movements:

➤ The Hundred

➤ Roll-Up

➤ Leg Circles

➤ Rolling Like a Ball

➤ Single-Leg Stretch

➤ Double-Leg Stretch

➤ Spine Stretch

➤ The Saw

➤ Side-Kick Series (turn to Chapter 11, "The Anticellulite Solution," for directions)

➤ Seal

You're striving to maintain good alignment:

➤ No belly bulging—keep scooping, scooping, scooping.

➤ No strain in the neck.

➤ No jerky movements in your body.

➤ No movement in your trunk—keep yourself anchored to the Mat.

➤ And finally, take deep breaths to empty your lungs completely.

➤ No looking up at the ceiling—eyes on your belly the whole time.

➤ No hunching your shoulders—shoulders are back and down, reaching long with your fingertips.

The message is clear: Take it slow. Yes, it's these small, specific goals that make it easier for you to achieve the bigger goal. Think of these first two weeks as a beginner class. As the weeks continue, you'll progress to an intermediate class by adding more exercises, each with a different focus and degree of difficulty. For now, stick to learning these exercises; it's the solid foundation for more stuff to come later. Keep at it, and within a few weeks you'll see a body line change that will not only make you feel good about what you've learned, but that also will dare you to show off your new bod!

Strike a Stance: The Pilates "V"

Strike a stance by gluing your heels together to make a small "V." Your feet are about three fingers apart. The legs slightly turn out, which begins in the hip bone socket and continues down the length of the legs to finish with your toes.

This "V" stabilizes your lower body, plus works some of the most neglected muscles—the back of your upper inner thighs! Joseph Pilates used to say, "Squeeze the backs of the upper inner thighs."

Be careful—don't turn out from the knees. This could throw off the alignment of your knee, foot, and ankle. To get a better feel, turn your leg in a parallel position, with the knee facing the ceiling—notice the straight alignment of the hip, knee, ankle, and foot? When you turn out, maintain this same integrity. Still, you shouldn't feel any stress in the knee or ankle joints. If you feel any pain, then look at your turnout because it may be too much.

Strive to keep this small "V" position with the heels glued together during all the moves.

Wake Up Your Body with the Hundred

Here's your warm-up, the Hundred. This move is a signature exercise developed by Joseph Pilates to warm up the body, preparing it for more to come. Regardless of the workout, the Hundred comes first to coordinate your breaths along with movement, increase circulation, and stabilize and warm up your core. Think of your lungs as a sponge—squeeze out the dirty water on the exhale so that the fresh water can enter.

You'll pump your arms about 6 to 8 inches, while inhaling for five counts and exhaling for five counts, adding up to 10 pumps of one complete breath. You'll pump for a grand total of 100 pumps, hence "the Hundred." During the pumping, nothing moves except your arms. If you don't have the core strength, your back may bounce off the floor as you pump. Think about the core concept: Anchor your spine to the Mat to stabilize your trunk.

Still, your neck may tire before your body does. This strain happens because of the combination of weak neck muscles, along with overtensing the neck muscles in the front as you fight to hold your head up. You can put one hand behind your head to support or lower your head to the Mat. Or, cut the pumps and breaths down to 50—quality versus quantity always. If you can't inhale for five, then reduce the breath counts. For example, start with two inhalations and exhale for two, and then progress to three and three.

Pilates Precaution

Don't turn out the feet too much. This can put too much stress on the knee and ankle joints. It's a forced movement that should be reserved only for dancers. If you have had any problems with sciatica, check with your doctor before turning out your legs. More than likely, you should not turn out your legs; work the legs in parallel instead.

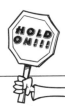

Pilates Precaution

Attention all beginners! For your first several sessions, always remember to keep your limbs close to your center. Make no big movements, and do fewer reps for quality over quantity.

Pump to the Hundred with this exercise:

1. Lie flat on your back with your arms by your sides, palms down.

2. Straighten your legs so that your toes reach out to a 45° angle or are in line with your eyes. If you feel your back lifting from the Mat, then raise your legs to the ceiling to maintain an anchored spine.

3. Hover your hands about 8 inches off the Mat, keeping them close to your body, palms down. Shoulders touch the Mat, and fingertips are reaching long, pits to your hip.

4. Inhale and vigorously pump your arms up and down for five counts, as if the arms are pumping through Jell-O, resisting each pump.

5. Exhale the air as you scoop your navel in and up. Imagine pasting your abs to your spine every time you exhale.

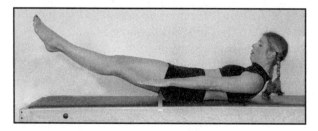

Modify the Hundred with this exercise:

1. Lie flat on your back, with your arms by your sides, palms down.

2. Pull one knee into your chest, and then pull in the other, keeping them close to your center. Lift your chin to your chest, and then begin pumping your arms.

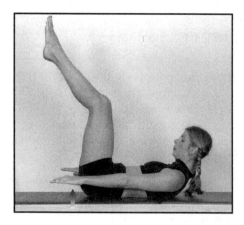

Roll-Up

Introducing the Roll-Up—it strengthens your powerhouse, plus keeps your spine flexible. A *happy joint* is a well-lubricated joint. The Roll-Up increases the *synovial fluids* throughout your spine as you roll up one vertebra at a time.

Remember peeling your spine off the Mat in the mini-exercise, imprinting? The same concept applies here. In the Roll-Up, peel your spine off the Mat, scooping the navel to the spine the whole time. Imagine lifting a string of pearls, one pearl at a time. That's how your spine will peel off the Mat, bone by bone.

Watch out for clenched shoulders on rolldown; relax and let them hang. No jerks up and plops down—use powerhouse control as you curl up and down. If you find that you can't control the roll, then try this: Bend your knees so that your hands can guide you up and down, or wrap a towel or Theraband around the front of your calves. Use the ends of the towel to guide you up and down.

Still, relax the quadriceps; instead work in your "V" and squeeze the backs of the inner thighs. You can imagine layers of Saran Wrap "wrapping" your hips together. This wrap will be used over and over again.

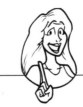

Pilates Lingo

A **happy joint** is a well-lubricated joint. Think of **synovial fluids** as WD-40 for your joints. When you move, especially in a slow, controlled manner, you're increasing synovial fluid production, whether it's in the spine, the hip, or the shoulder. This keeps your joints flexible, protects them from seizing up, and perhaps prevents one of today's most debilitating diseases—arthritis.

Roll up like a wheel in motion in these steps:

1. Lie flat on your back in the Pilates "V," with your feet flexed.

2. Raise your arms over your head in the frame of your body, dropping your rib cage, spine to Mat.

3. Inhale and bring your chin to your chest to initiate the Roll-Up. Press your heels away from your hips, and squeeze the backs of the upper thighs to control the Roll-Up. Fingertips reach long, while your ears remain between your upraised arms.

4. Exhale as the fingers reach long past your toes, and scoop even more.

5. Inhale to initiate the 6–12 pelvic curl to scoop and roll down to the middle of your back, pinching your butt-cheeks. Press your heels away from your hips, and squeeze the backs of your upper thighs.

6. Exhale to roll your spine down the Mat, bone by bone. Repeat five times, as if you're a wheel in motion.

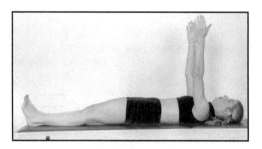
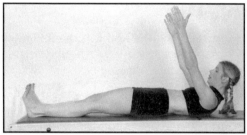
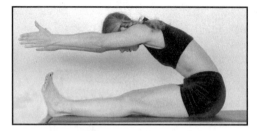
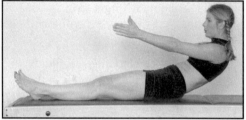

Flex and Stretch: Hamstrings, Ankles, Leg Circles

After the Roll-Up, stretch the hamstrings group to warm up the leg for the next exercise, Leg Circles. The hamstrings are a group of muscles in the back of the leg that flex and bend the knee. The problem is, many of us either neglect this group or sit all day. As a result, the hamstrings shorten and tighten.

Shortened tight hamstrings can affect the position of the pelvis, which could eventually lead to poor posture.

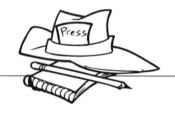

Pilates Scoop

If you allow your abdomen to bulge like a loaf of bread, then you are no longer using your abdominal muscles correctly. Remember, transform your transverse. The abs are in and up under the rib cage—scoop, scoop, scoop.

Stretching the hamstrings can alleviate some of the tightness. As always, stay anchored so that your sacrum touches the floor. Don't arch your neck or lift your head off the floor. Relax the shoulders. If you can't reach behind your leg or your calf, then wrap a towel over the sole of your foot. Grab the ends of the towel so that you can stretch the leg correctly. Don't grab behind the knee or lift your hip off the Mat, thinking that the stretch will increase. To stretch the hamstrings, you have to square off your hips:

1. Inhale to prepare for the stretch.
2. Exhale to pull your belly in and up, and slowly pull your leg toward your face. Press your butt bones to the floor, and reach your heels out of your hips for control and to increase the stretch.

3. Pause. Release the stretch. Repeat three times, and then perform a series of ankle circles.

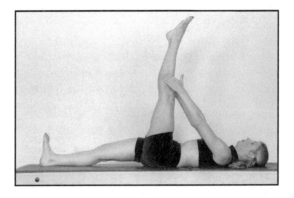

Ankle Circles

Let's give the ankles some attention. Foot circles warm up the ankle joints, increase flexibility, and stretch some of the lower leg muscles. Between lugging heavy bones and wearing tight, constricting shoes, your ankles never seem to get a break. After the hamstring stretch, circle your ankles. Roll outward five times, and then reverse the direction, inward for five circles. Imagine this: You're splashing your feet in a pool of beach water and, as you slowly circle, the sand runs through your toes.

Don't forget about your often neglected toes. Flex the foot by pushing your heel away from your face, and softly point energy out of the big toe. Flex and point three times.

Leg Circles

All this prep was to warm up your legs for Leg Circles. You'll circle the leg to challenge your trunk. Remember, movement of the limbs initiates from the core-trunk-torso! Still, Leg Circles warm up the hips and joints, plus tighten and tone areas that can't be hidden by a bathing suit: abs, thighs, and hips.

The hip joint is a ball-and-socket joint; it has the ability to move in a wide range of movements. You can stir, kick, and circle your leg. Try this: Bring your knee into your chest. Gently press the bones of the hip until you feel the bone in its joint. If you can't feel this, stir the knee in tiny circles as if you're stirring a thick soup. Do you feel the head of the *femur*, your thigh bone, move inside its socket?

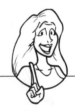

Pilates Lingo

Whenever you read **bone in its joint**, that means that the joint is in its proper place. This proper joint alignment permits the limbs to move safely in a wide variety of movements without wear and tear on the joint. Bone in its joint particularly pertains to the ball-and-socket joints of the hip and shoulder joints. Remember, first you stabilize the body, and then you move it!

As you circle the leg, this bone moves within the joint, reducing stress on the joint. You'll always work with the *bone in its joint*; you will always stabilize the body before moving it.

You have two goals: Stabilize the pelvis and prevent the hips from rocking side to side as the leg circles. To do this, press the palms of your hands, the back of your head, and the back of your arms into the Mat to brace a very heavy torso at all times. Also, keep the circles small at first (as shown in the accompanying pictures). Imagine a string looped around your big toe; it's pulling your toe to the ceiling so that the up-lifted leg is straight. If you can't straighten the uplifted leg, then bend the knee softly.

1. Lie flat on your back, pressing the base of your head and the back of your arms into the Mat, palms down.

2. Raise one leg up to the ceiling, slightly turning out from the hip, with your leg in line with your nose.

3. Inhale to lift your leg to the nose and take the leg across the body; your hips can lift slightly.

4. Exhale to take the leg down toward the Mat, keeping your trunk stable and out to the side. Then inhale your leg up to your nose, stopping on a dime with a slight pause.

5. Repeat five circles, and then reverse. Repeat the whole sequence on the other leg: hamstring, ankle, circles.

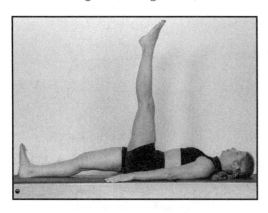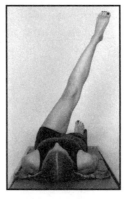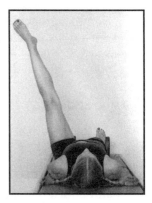

Rolling Like a Ball

Get ready for a spine treat. You're rolling to ease spinal tension, add balance work, and discover how to control your momentum in the roll itself. Momentum is typically a no-no, but in rolling, you'll use core concepts to control the momentum and increase the intensity: 6–12 curl to secure your scoop and pinch your butt cheeks together.

To get in position, sit at the edge of the Mat. Slide your bottom to your heels. Place the palms of your hands behind your thighs, and practice the 6–12 curl, scooping your navel. Try scooping so much that your toes lift off the ground. Now, actually lift your toes up so that they hover about 2 to 3 inches off the ground. You might lose your 6–12 curl here but deeply scoop to control the wobble.

To roll with ease at first, you can open your knees slightly or touch your toes to the Mat if you feel super wobbly. However, to progress, you need to focus on pinching your butt cheeks as well as scooping to roll without momentum. In the roll, the shoulders will have a tendency to creep toward your ears—de-hunch them. And here's the important part: chin to chest so that you look at your belly button the whole time.

Do wobble-free rolls with these steps:

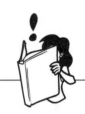

1. Wrap your right hand over your left ankle, while the left hand crosses the right wrist. Your heels stay close to your bottom.

2. Lower your head so that your eyes are on your belly, chin to chest. The head will never touch the Mat. Don't scrunch the spine; it's a lift up and over!

3. Inhale as you roll back, pinch your butt cheeks, scoop your belly, and lift your tailbone to the ceiling. Stay tight.

4. Exhale as you roll up, and scoop your belly to protect your lower back—no belly bulge.

5. Repeat 8 to 10 times, keeping the motion going.

Pilates Primer

Among Pilates's brilliant moves is Rolling Like a Ball. The "rolling" is a good example of driving out the impurities. As you roll and unroll your spine—vertebra by vertebra—you're cleansing the lungs.

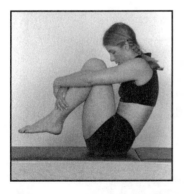
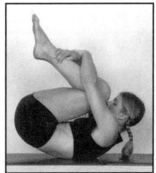
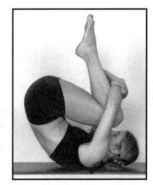

Single- and Double-Leg Stretch

The warm-up is over! You're now increasing the intensity: The Single-Leg Stretch uses 100 percent pure abs. This stretch initiates a series of ab exercises known as the "fives." You'll do the "twos," however. Like the Hundred, these exercises coordinate breath and ab work as you move your limbs and stabilize the torso, requiring a great deal of coordination and concentration.

Single-Leg Stretch

So, where's the stretch? Imagine your leg stretching for miles and miles—1, 2, 3 miles long as the big toe lengthens away from the hips. The toe is in line with the nose; pinch your butt cheeks, and use those thighs! Your neck may tire first, so make sure that your chin is on your chest and that your eyes look at your navel the whole time; lower your head, however, if you feel any neck strain. Don't stop the exercise, though. Lift your head into position after a little rest.

Start your intense ab work with the Single-Leg Stretch:

1. Anchor your spine to the Mat. Bring your knees into your chest. At the same time, stretch your left leg so that your toe is in line with your nose; place your right hand on the outside of the right ankle or near it, while your left hand rests on the inside of your right knee, elbows wide. This hand position keeps your knee aligned with the ankle, knee, and hip.

2. Lift your chin to your chest, and stretch the left leg long, softly pointing the toes, a couple inches off the Mat or higher, depending where you can anchor the spine. Inhale gradually for two leg stretches.

3. Exhale as you switch your legs and lengthen away from the hips for two stretches. Blow all the air out of your lungs to flatten your belly. Pull your left leg in to your chest as the right foot lengthens long. Keep your leg high to secure your back to the Mat, if needed. As your core strength improves, you'll skim the Mat with your toes.

4. Repeat four to eight stretches, with eight stretches per leg.

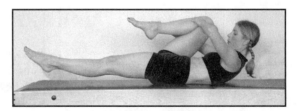

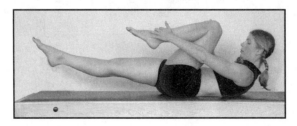

Double-Leg Stretch

Rest for a minute, and then continue this ab series with the Double-Leg Stretch. As your core strength develops, you won't need to rest. In addition to developing your core, you're testing your coordination and endurance.

Up the ab work with these steps:

1. Recheck your body. If you need to anchor your spine, do so.

2. Draw your knees into your chest. Place your hands on your shins. Keep your chin on your chest, and scoop your belly.

3. Press your legs, if you can, into your chest to blow all the air out. Inhale to extend all four limbs to the ceiling—or out to a 45° angle, depending on your ability to anchor your spine. At no time should you arch your back; keep a firm and stable trunk.

4. Exhale and gracefully circle the arms, with your hands toward the ceiling and then behind your head, stretching your fingers long over your head. At the same time, reach your toes long. The arms move a second or two before the legs. The legs follow the arms into the chest to the start position. The trunk never moves!

5. Repeat five smooth, flowing stretches.

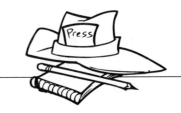

Pilates Scoop

If you find that your belly muscles are outlasting your neck, then you have a few options: Put one hand behind your head, place your hands on your thighs and extend them, or lower your head to the floor. If you still feel that the exercise is too stressful, use a small pillow to support your head and neck.

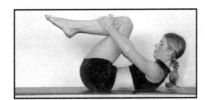

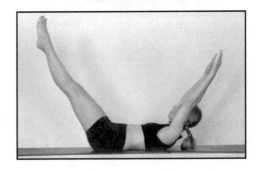

Spine Stretch

Finally, a stretch. You've earned it after all that hard abdominal work. Let's stretch the spine and the hamstrings, plus reinforce your commitment to stacking the spine bone by bone. During this stretch, make sure that you empty your lungs and inhale. Remember, your lungs are like a sponge!

1. Sit on the Mat with your legs spread a little more than shoulder width.

2. Anchor your butt bones to the Mat. Pinch, lift, and grow tall. Remain committed to your scoop, in and up.

3. Flex your toes so that you feel a stretch in the hamstrings, but don't lock your knees. Inhale into your back.

4. Exhale and lower your chin to your chest, and curl the top of your head toward the floor, scooping the whole time. Aim your nose toward your tailbone.

5. At the same time, stretch your fingertips, extending past an imaginary line running between your feet. Even though your arms are stretching forward, keep scooping your navel to your spine. When you've stretched to your limits, pause.

6. Inhale into your back to restack your spine while pressing the back of your legs into the Mat to secure your bottom.

7. Repeat five times, even though you'll be tempted to do more.

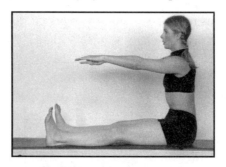

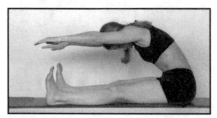

The Saw

Joseph Pilates said, "Wring out the lungs like a dish towel." In his exercise the Saw, you'll twist your torso to wring out the lungs of all their impurities; it's a waist-trimming exercise that also stretches the hamstrings.

Imagine the belly button lifting and then twisting the torso as you reach for the little toe to saw it off. Focus on the up and over.

Saw in these steps:

1. Sit on the Mat with your legs straight out in front of you, a little wider than shoulder width.

2. Anchor your heels and butt bones to the Mat, and scoop. Raise your arms straight out at your sides, and pull them apart, palms down and reaching your fingertips long. Inhale to grow tall and, lift your ribs off your pelvis and initiate the twist.

3. Exhale deeper into the twist. Imagine your navel twisting your torso as your right hand reaches past your left foot, as if sawing off your pinky toe. Your ear listens to your knee as you look behind to twist a little farther, each time exhaling every ounce of air out of your lungs; it's not a bounce.

4. To get the most of this stretch, reach your left hand behind you, turning your palm up. Inhale and return to the starting position even taller—pinch, lift, and grow! Exhale to twist the other way.

5. Repeat three to four sets.

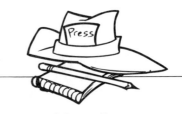

Pilates Scoop

To sit up out of your hips, visualize your head floating up, up, up to the clouds. Use the inner thighs, lower tush, and belly to help create length all the way up the spine. If you're collapsing in your hips, meaning that you can't sit up out of your hips, then place a small pad under your butt.

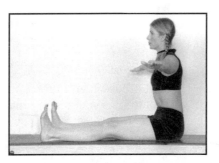

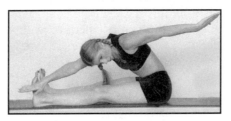

Seal

Bark like a seal; and clap your heels together. Sound suspicious? That's how you'll end Mat. What's the point? It's fun, relieves tension in your spine, and works on balance and control. This clap comes from the hips, not the feet, to make the powerhouse work. At first, clap in front. As you advance, you can clap in both directions, in front and overhead.

1. Wrap your arms under your legs, reaching under your knees, outside your ankles, to grab your feet.

2. Heels together—clap your heels and bark like a seal. Just warming up! Scoop and look at your belly the whole time. Take a breath!

3. Exhale and roll back, lifting your butt cheeks in the air—pinching the entire time—until your weight shifts to your shoulder blades. Your head never touches the floor. For the advanced, clap while balancing on your shoulder blades.

4. Inhale to roll up, scooping your belly; focus on your navel. Balance and clap your heels together. Repeat 8 to 10 times.

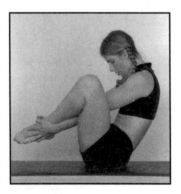 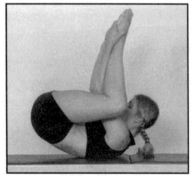

Wrapping It Up

The message is clear: Joseph Pilates rules. Even in the earlier stages, you can develop strength and flexibility in each muscle, work on coordination, and de-wobble your body. These exercises were perfectly arranged to give you a total body workout.

Try to commit these exercises to memory. As you see, the core concepts are used in every move, no matter what. Be kind to yourself if you feel a little uncoordinated or wobbly. The movements take time to penetrate your mind and body. You won't build strength overnight, so don't rush the movement or learning—quality over quantity. After all, you have a lifetime to enjoy the range of exercises and benefits. Relax, stick with it, and scoop, scoop, scoop!

The Least You Need to Know

➤ Glue your heels and thighs together; toes are about 3 inches apart to strike a Pilates "V."

➤ Do the exercises in order, because that's how Joseph Pilates arranged them to work the muscles symmetrically.

➤ Layer the moves to build a solid foundation; it's these small, specific goals that make it easy to achieve the bigger goal.

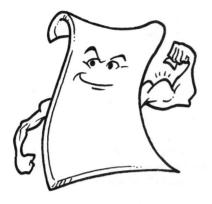

Chapter 7

Get the Man-Made Mat Body

In This Chapter

➤ You'll never do a crunch again

➤ Recommit to your scoop

➤ Learn the principles of overload

➤ Strong and long

Great bodies are made, not born: It's the subtle curves of the thigh, the rippling of the abs, the lift in the derriere, and the sculpted arms that make a body good-looking.

So, how can you get a good-looking body? You have to create it yourself, and there's no way around it. For a sleek, strong, well-toned body, you have to move the body a new way and add resistance to your workout. You must challenge the muscles even if you're devoted to your workout.

Your goal is to activate more muscle fibers: Go slow, hold the body a little longer, squeeze each muscle, and challenge your muscles with a little extra body weight.

The results? A man-made bod!

Busting Your Gut

So crunches didn't work for you? Don't worry; you're not alone. Join the ranks of the millions who crunched their bellies into a big fat bulge. So, why did we do it? Perhaps it was to get rid of our back pain. We've heard that strong abs can lessen the workload of your back muscles, which is true. Or, maybe it was pure vanity; we wanted that rippled six-pack look. Whatever the reason, we crunched our heart out for nothing—a bulging potbelly. How discouraging! Don't settle for nil happening below the waist.

Traditionally, there's the crunch or a sit-up. Both abdominal exercises strengthen muscles, but not always your abs. Actually, instead of flattening your mid-appearance, you've probably given your hip flexors a workout. The major hip flexor muscle, *illiopsoas* (or psoas for short), starts in the crease of your upper thigh and wraps through the pelvis to attach to the lumbar vertebrae; it lifts your knee to your chest.

When you crunch, or do a sit-up, the psoas muscle responds probably more than your abs. Why? Because this muscle is often tight from overuse and strong from being overdeveloped, which can cause lower back pain in the end.

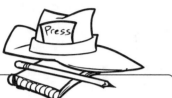

Pilates Scoop

If you're not positioning your body correctly when performing a crunch or sit-up, then you're creating a monster bulge in the belly rather than the sleek slender abs you so deserve.

Securing Your Scoop

If you "spring" up to do a sit-up or crunch, then either the psoas is tight from being overworked or you don't have the ab strength—perhaps a combination of both. Neither scenario is good because you'll probably feel this "spring" in your back. Let's say that you have a combination of strong hip flexors and weak abs, yet you're determined to do a sit-up. You'll get up; however, the tight shortened hip flexor responds by pulling the *lumbar vertebra* into play. When this happens, the lower back arches, which also naturally slightly bulges or distends the belly. Consequently, you'll feel a tug in your lower back.

If you continue to "situp" or "crunch" without securing your scoop, you'll end up with a combination of weak abs, even tighter psoas, and a bigger muscle monster bulge. Try it for yourself.

To sit up, crunch, or roll the spine into an upright position safely, you need less hip flexors and more abdominal strength. To do this, you must maintain a neutral pelvis and simply scoop! And that's one reason why the Roll-Up is such an effective midsection reducer and core strengthener.

First, you anchor the spine and scoop your belly button before any movement; it's called centering. Not only does this position flatten your belly, but it also protects your back. Second, you're told to keep the head in line with the spine the whole time!

Finally, you peel your spine off the Mat, bone by bone. The movement, then, becomes a slow and controlled movement rather than a series of "spring-ups."

The Strong and Long

Elongation during the entire movement, through full range of motion, is a must to create the long and strong body! We've been conditioned to believe that it takes mega-reps with lots of weight to build muscle strength. That's not always the case, though. In fact, if the muscle tires, it works in a contracted or shortened length. Muscles can work easier in a contracted state, so what you're really developing is strength and bulge.

Your muscles contract three ways: *isometrically, concentrically,* and *eccentrically.* If you work without balance between the muscle groups, then imbalance happens. Concentric contraction shortens the muscles as it contracts; for example, a biceps curl shortens the biceps muscle. If you reverse the direction, then you're lengthening the muscle, which is an eccentric contraction. Isometric contractions hold the muscle in place to create a static muscle contraction.

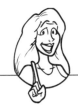

Pilates Lingo

Concentric contraction shortens the muscle, while **eccentric contraction** lengthens the muscle. For example, do a bicep curl, and you're shortening the muscle. Reverse the curl, and now you're lengthening the muscle. An isometric contraction means that the muscle doesn't move when it's contracted.

If you're not lengthening the muscle by working in a full range of motion, then you're shortening the muscle. Not to pick on the "crunch" again; however, this abdominal exercise provides the perfect example of how we shorten a muscle. Here's why: The emphasis is to bend forward—crunch, crunch, crunch. You're shortening and strengthening the most superficial abdominal muscle, the rectus, because the muscle doesn't reach its full length on the way down. Reasons for muscles not reaching full length vary: The muscle can be tired, you're not practicing good form, the emphasis is on the shortened contraction, and the movements can be fast and out-of-control.

It's easier to work the muscles short as in a crunch. You probably can do fifty crunches, but doing five Roll-Ups is another story. Why? Because the focus is to work all the abdominal muscles (rectus, transversus, internal and external obliques) evenly, and in a full range of motion. If you don't lengthen and work the abdominals evenly, then you get muscle imbalances—hence, muscle monster!

You won't be able to do many reps of these exercises. The emphasis is full range of motion to lengthen the muscles—plus, you work for muscle symmetry, which is why these exercises tend to be a physical challenge even if you can bench-press a car!

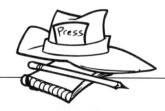

Pilates Scoop

Go ahead crunch your heart out. You might have nothing to show for it except a big, fat belly bulge. Crunches work the abdominals by shortening the muscles, not lengthening them. This one-sided contraction creates a muscle imbalance, plus the focus is to develop the rectus muscles. This, too, creates an imbalance between the muscle groups, which can contribute to a bulging belly look. You have to work the muscles evenly and in full range of motion to change your look.

Corkscrews, Swans, and Neck Pulls, Oh My!

Okay, you got it; the moves are more challenging. You need to return to the guiding principle: control. The emphasis for these two weeks is to engage even more muscle fibers and to crank up the brain power to make your body move the way you want it to, with control.

The new moves are these: Open Leg Rocker, the Swan, Single-Leg Kick, Corkscrew, Neck Pull, and Side-Kick Series for weeks 3 and 4. You're moving away from the introductory work to advance your workout. For example, after you've completed the Spine Stretch, add the Open-Leg Rocker. After that, you'll do the Corkscrew, the Saw, and so forth. You're building your Mat workout, so practice the moves that you've already learned. Here's how these exercises fit into the program to develop your body uniformly:

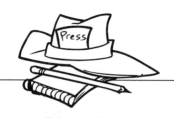

Pilates Scoop

Do the exercises in order. There is a definite progression: Each move prepares you for the next, which is more challenging. Joseph Pilates brilliantly masterminded each move to work each muscle, without fatigue and strain.

➤ The Hundred
➤ Roll-Up
➤ Leg Circles
➤ Rolling Like a Ball
➤ Single-Leg Stretch
➤ Double-Leg Stretch
➤ Spine Stretch
➤ Open-Leg Rocker
➤ Corkscrew 1
➤ The Saw

➤ Single-Leg Kick

➤ Swan 1

➤ Neck Pull

➤ Side-Kick Series (see Chapter 11, "The Anticellulite Solution")

➤ Seal

Open-Leg Rocker

Can you balance? Can you stay in control? The Open-Leg Rocker tests how complete you are. Finding imbalances in your body is a good thing. We may have a tendency to roll to one side if that side is stronger than the other. The goal is to roll evenly to balance the muscles of the spine and abdominals; work them as a team to roll with balance and control.

You must scoop, scoop, scoop. The Open-Leg Rocker is 100 percent belly! Keep your center firm, scooping harder and harder to control the roll. Remember, squeeze every ounce of air out to protect your lower back.

Go for advanced Open-Leg Rocker in these steps:

1. Sit on the Mat. Roll your pelvis into a 6–12 curl to balance. The legs lift up to the ceiling to create a "V," and feet are at eye level. The legs are a little wider than your shoulders. All limbs are straight, and your chin is on your chest.

2. Inhale to roll back, making sure that your weight lands on your shoulders and that your head never touches the Mat.

3. Exhale to roll up, and scoop to a balanced "V" position. If you come up too quickly or flop to one side, then slightly bend your knees and tighten your tummy—it's all about focus, balance, and control. Repeat five times.

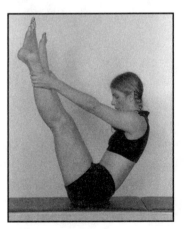 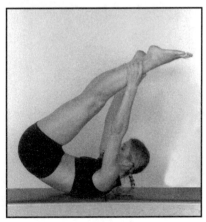

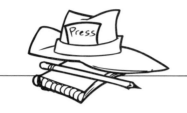

Pilates Scoop

The Open-Leg Rocker is a great exercise that tests your coordination and strength, as well as your flexibility and control in motion. You may find muscle imbalances between the left and right sides of your body. The goal is to roll evenly to balance the muscles of the spine and abdominals; work them as a team to roll with balance and control.

Modify the Open-Leg Rocker with these steps:

1. Get in position and wrap your arms underneath the legs to lift your knees up; toes should dangle just off the Mat.

2. Inhale as you lift your left leg, with your toes reaching to the ceiling. Don't round your back, yet stay steady in your pelvis.

3. Exhale and lower your left leg. Inhale and lift your right leg. Again, focus on scooping to help stabilize your pelvis. Exhale and lower your right leg. Do three reps.

4. Inhale to straighten both legs to a "V." Exhale to close the "V," and inhale to reopen the "V." Exhaling lowers the legs to the floor.

5. Try this exercise four times.

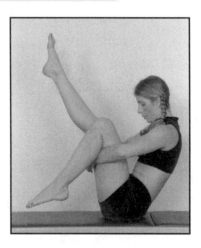 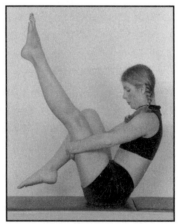

The Corkscrew

The Corkscrew strengthens the deep abs while challenging your trunk stability as you circle your legs as if they were one. The limbs move from the core, so you must center before circling the legs.

There are a few versions of the Corkscrew; here, however, you'll see only one.

Focus on firmness up and down the spine. The tendency is to arch the neck or back off the Mat as the weight of the legs circle down. Anchor from the base of your head to your sacrum, and press the backs of your arms into the Mat, palms down.

Do the Corkscrew in these steps:

1. Anchor from the back of your neck to the base of your spine to the Mat. Your hands should be by your side, pressing palms into the Mat for stability. The shoulders are back and down, pits to your hips.

2. Raise your legs to the ceiling. Imagine a string pulling your toes to the ceiling, so lengthen the legs away from the hips, keeping your knees and ankles together.

3. Inhale to make a small circle with the legs to the left, leading with your big toe and letting the right hip come off the Mat slightly. Keep your knees and ankles together the entire time.

4. Exhale to complete the circle. Then reverse—circle right and finish left. Keep the circle small, to prevent you from lifting your back and neck off the Mat. Repeat three to five times.

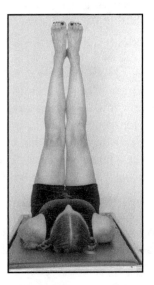 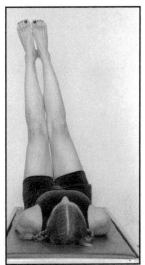

Take Flight with the Swan

Flip over; it's time to work the backside. Up to this point, you have worked mostly in a forward flexion, meaning abs on fire! Now, it's time to stretch the abs and work the spine. In other words, you're working your body in the opposite direction. But your abs still must work a little—in fact, they must work eccentrically to lengthen your look. Remember the core concepts threaded throughout all the exercises, no matter what position you're in. And this is for stability against movement! Therefore, even if you're on your belly, scoop the navel into the spine.

If you keep in mind the natural progression of the spine, then you can redevelop the muscles, stabilize the body correctly, and perform the exercises safely. The tendency is to let the front side hang, giving no support to the delicate muscles along your spine and abdominals. The shoulders tend to hunch toward the ears.

It's the same core concepts; you're just using them in a different direction: Lift the navel to the spine, and pinch your butt cheeks to hold a thousand-dollar bill so that you activate your pelvic floor muscles, the back of your upper thighs, and on down. Your shoulders are back and down, drawing the shoulder blades down your back. Every muscle must work, including your powerhouse.

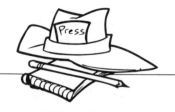

Pilates Scoop

Extension always starts with the head, and then the body will follow.

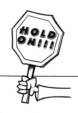

Pilates Precaution

Be careful—it's not a face drop. Don't give your dentist any more business by knocking out your two front teeth. Control your rocks by pushing and pulling with the palms of your hands, and keep your elbows glued to your rib cage.

In the prep, you'll just lift the torso and roll the head to one side and then the other. This move will help you gain strength in the muscles in the back and abs, while stretching the neck muscles.

Take flight with the Swan in these steps:

1. Lie on your stomach.

2. Place your hands directly under your shoulders, palms down. Elbows are close to your rib cage. Stretch your toes long, as if a string is pulling on your big toe. Put some tone in your butt cheeks, lift up your navel, and press your shoulders back and down to your hips.

3. Inhale and slowly lift your breastbone to the ceiling, as if you're a skittish turtle not wanting to come out of your shell. Create length in the back of your neck to the base of the spine, keeping your shoulders down.

4. Keep lifting as you look at the wall—as long as you can—while pushing your palms into the Mat. Think up, up, up as not to crush the vertebra; pinch, pinch, pinch the butt cheeks. Brush your rib cage with your elbows. Keep them close to your body as the shoulder blades descend down your back.

5. Exhale, drop your torso, and lift the legs at the same time, keeping the elbows by your side to control the dive. The palms of your hands support the weight of your trunk. Keep your face up, and stay lifted. It doesn't have to be a big drop; just get used to rocking from front to back.

6. Repeat three to five times.

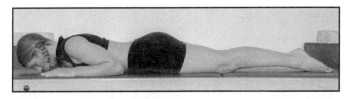

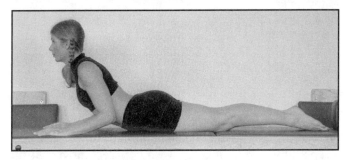

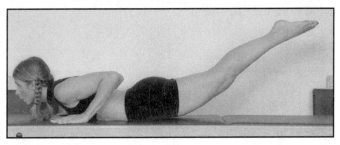

Single-Leg Kick

Stay on your backside, lifting your abs and working the muscles along your spine. It's time for the Single-Leg Kick, which actually stretches the quads while you strengthen the hamstrings and gluteus. The Single-Leg Kick is also a coordination exercise because you alternate the legs as they "kick-pulse" from left to right. Same rules apply. Put an imaginary thousand-dollar bill between your butt cheeks and squeeze, and press your thigh bones into the Mat.

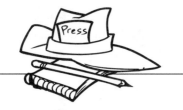

Pilates Scoop

Single-Leg Kicks are snappy kicks that test your coordination. Keep kicking to establish a nice rhythm from left to right, never setting your leg down before the other leg is up—kick and pulse. Don't let the thigh bones shift from side to side—no dancing hips.

To modify this exercise, you can put a pillow underneath your belly to help support your back. If you feel any pressure in the knees, then put a towel or pad underneath to cushion them.

Here's what you need to do:

1. Lie on the Mat and lift your abs.

2. Squeeze your butt cheeks, and press your thigh bones into the Mat. Put your elbows directly under your shoulders and toward the belly to make an upside-down "V." Press your elbows into the Mat.

3. Make a fist, and put your hands together. Lift your head out of your shoulders as your breastbone lifts to the ceiling so that it lengthens away from the hips.

4. Inhale and draw your right heel to your butt, keeping your trunk secure.

5. Pump rapidly—kick and pulse, keeping your knee pressing into the Mat.

6. As you return the heel to the Mat, exhale and bring the left heel up—kick and pulse. Keep a steady rhythm going, with both legs moving at the same time. Guess what's not moving—your pelvis. No dancing hips, and no butt-cheek jiggle.

7. Do three to five sets.

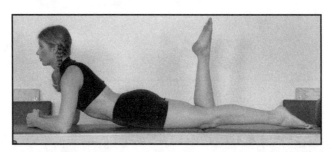

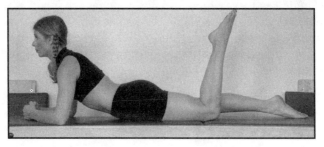

The Much-Needed Rest: Child's Pose

Your spine muscles need a rest now. Get in a position called Child's Pose, and inhale and exhale after oh-so-much work. There's nothing to it. Breathe naturally, in and out five times or so. Imagine your spine collapsing with every deep exhalation, releasing the grippers or tight muscles in the spine; just let your body wind down.

Relax in Child's Pose with these steps:

1. Slide your bottom back so that it's resting on your heels. Arms go over your head or down by your side.

2. Inhale up into your spine, and exhale to pull the belly off the thighs.

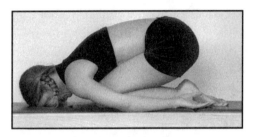

Back to the Belly: Neck Pull

Okay, back to work. Let's finish with the Neck Pull; it's another belly exercise that makes you sweat.

The good news is, you'll use the same core concepts: peeling your spine bone by bone, anchoring your spine to the Mat, putting your chin to your chest, pinching your butt cheeks, and so forth. However, the Neck Pull challenges the powerhouse even more. For this exercise, imagine curling and uncurling your spine like you're opening a can of sardines.

Here's a warning: If you feel pulling in your back, start with the bent knee modification. In other words, you'll do the same steps, only with your knees bent. Take your time with this exercise; it's definitely a gut challenge—but not at the risk to your back, please.

Fire up the abs with the Neck Pull in these steps:

1. Anchor your spine to the Mat, and scoop.

2. Hands clasps behind your head, with your elbows on the Mat to see them from your peripheral vision. Open your legs so that they are about hip-width apart. Press your heels away from your hips.

3. Inhale to lift your chin to your chest, and peel your spine off the Mat, and scoop. Don't hide your face as you roll up; your elbows are in your peripheral vision.

4. Exhale as you curl your nose to your belly button. Remember, glue the abs to your spine!

5. Inhale to stack your bones as you uncurl your head to the ceiling until you're sitting out of your hips.

6. Still inhaling, lean back into a plank position so that your stomach is flat, with your heels pressing away from your hips. Pinch your butt cheeks to keep you stable.

7. Exhale as you go into a 6–12 curl to roll down bone by bone. Keep your abs as close to your back as possible, press your heels away from your hips, and squeeze your butt cheeks.

8. Press your heels away as you roll down bone by bone until the very last vertebra is between your ears. Don't plop down!

9. Repeat three to five times.

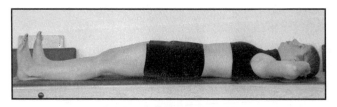

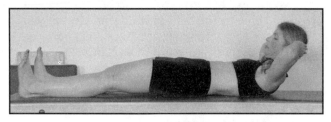

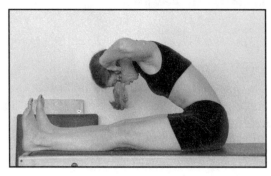

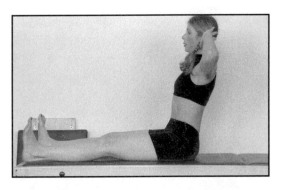

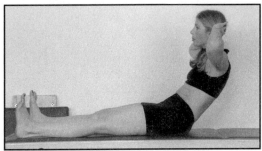

It's a Wrap

After week 4, you should definitely witness a shift. Perhaps you can almost fit into your favorite pair of jeans, or the love handles are diminishing. Maybe you just feel great because you're doing something wonderful for your body. Oh yeah, squeeze, squeeze, squeeze!

The Least You Need to Know

➤ To change your body, you'll need to go slow, hold the body a little longer, and squeeze each muscle.

➤ You're creating a bulging monster if you do crunches only.

➤ Pilates's exercises work the body in a full range of motion, emphasizing an eccentric contraction to create the long and strong body.

➤ Extension always starts with the head, and then the body will follow.

➤ Use the breath to move the body.

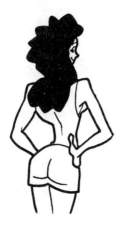

Chapter 8

Graduate to the "It" Body

In This Chapter

➤ Love-handle-free—and loving life

➤ Connect the moves with transitions

➤ Increase intensity with more challenging moves

➤ Seven new moves to complete the shape-up basics

If you've got it, flaunt it. But what if you lost it along the way? Can you still get it? Chiseling your curves so that you can show off your body is what these last two weeks brings you. Getting the body that you want may simply be a matter of taking the moves you've been doing one step further.

To get the "it" body, you must turn up the heat. You'll work in several new positions to recruit more muscle as you challenge your body in a few different planes of movement. You'll use your body in big movements to create even more resistance for your core and limbs.

Consider your body a temple; its parts work flawlessly to move in harmony so that you can flaunt it.

Flaunting Your Flow

To keep your body primed, you must increase the degree of difficulty—you know this already. So, in these weeks, you'll incorporate the overload principle of time. In fact, you'll reduce your workout time by moving through the exercises a little faster, yet never sacrificing good form. And how? By focusing on the guiding principle of flow.

Think of your workout as one big dance, with movements connecting from one to another by way of a transitional move. In weeks 5 and 6, you've advanced to intermediate status. You should have exercises committed to memory: the order, exercise, breathing patterns, and how to safely move. Running through them without stopping is icing on the cake; it's fine-tuning.

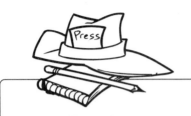

Pilates Scoop

If these moves are too easy, re-evaluate your form. Even in weeks 5 and 6, you should be very challenged by the exercises themselves. In addition, you're striving to embody the guiding principle: flow. You will flow from one move to another; flow transfers into your daily life in the way of grace!

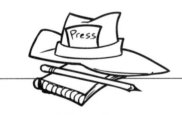

Pilates Scoop

Pilates trains you for life and makes you stronger for everyday movements. It improves your flexibility, coordination, muscle strength, and muscle stamina. Can you think of ways in your everyday life that require you to move in so many training modes?

Imagine that you're an Olympic competitor going for the gold. It's not enough just to know the routine. There's that something extra that distinguishes between the gold and silver medals. You're focused, executing each move with precision and control, and your routine just flows. That's your goal for these weeks: Allow no wasted motion. Come prepared to perform, to show off your stuff.

Here's the transition rule: If your legs finish on the floor—let's say, after Leg Circles—then do a Roll-Up to the next move, which would be Rolling Like a Ball. As another example, after you complete the Fives, then do a Roll-Up to get in position for the Spine Stretch.

Ready, Set, Rhythm?

Have you ever tapped your foot as a song plays on the radio? That's rhythm! It's a regular succession of moves that's difficult to put in words. But it's in your body, and inevitably it will be in your Mat.

Certain exercises are intended to click along at a succinct pace. Just like the rap-a-tap-tap of your toes, a few moves will spur a little soul in you. Take the Side-Kick Series, for example. One leg moves gracefully into the next move, into the next, and so forth. You keep the work flowing from leg exercise to leg exercise. While rhythm is often very individual and elusive, you'll get pointers on how to move from one exercise to the next, and you'll have fun doing so.

So, why rhythm? It's hard work, for one, and you're developing muscle stamina, meaning that you're training the muscle to work over and over again. A body builder, for example, will have muscle strength or the ability to lift heavy loads. Muscle stamina, though, is a more subtle strength. A boxer is a perfect example. The fact that he can throw a series of rapid-fire punches is muscle stamina. It's a way of upping the workload so that your body evolves stronger and more refined. In other words, it's details. Sure, you can memorize the moves, but it's the details that make the mind and body work in harmony. No move should be just a move!

If You've Got It, Flaunt It!

How will you improve your muscle endurance? Develop a balanced body? And refine your body? By asking your muscles to do more. The real challenge comes from integrating several muscle groups in nontraditional ways. Instead of working just forward and back, you'll stabilize the core while lifting a leg or an arm. After all, that's how we move in life. You squat and twist to pick something off the floor. There are no pure exercises—all involve several muscle groups, as well as stretching to keep the body nimble and healthy. You flex and stretch in every move. In a sense, these exercises prepare your muscles for how they work in your day-to-day life.

There's always a way to increase the intensity to keep your body primed and challenged.

In these weeks, you'll add more movement, use the guiding principle control to work the muscles instead of moving them with momentum, and use flow to eliminate the rest periods between exercises. You'll also attempt to establish a nice rhythm by completing the Fives and the Side-Kick Series. And you'll add these exercises: Double-Leg Kick, Swimming, Shoulder Bridge (stability), Leg Pulls (stability), and Teaser 1.

Remember, you're striving for efficiency and control, not speed and haphazard movements. Here's the entire sequence of exercises:

➤ The Hundred

➤ Roll-Up

➤ Leg Circles

➤ Rolling Like a Ball

➤ The Fives: Single-Leg Stretch, Double-Leg Stretch, Single Straight-Leg Stretch, Double Straight-Leg Stretch, and Crisscross

➤ Spine Stretch

➤ Open-Leg Rocker

➤ Corkscrew

➤ The Saw

➤ The Swan

➤ Single-Leg Kick

➤ Double-Leg Kick

➤ Neck Pull

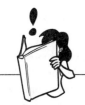

Pilates Primer

Joseph Pilates invented a variety of moves to develop the whole body and all its muscles. After all, that's how we move in real life.

➤ The Bridge (stabilize)

➤ Side-Kick Series (all)

➤ Teaser 1

➤ Swimming

➤ Leg Pull Front (stabilize)

➤ Leg Pull Back (stabilize)

➤ The Seal

Love-Handle-Free and Loving It: The Fives

Imagine the Energizer bunny—it just keeps going and going and going! So will your powerhouse. It works to stabilize your trunk while you lower, lift, and scissor the legs. Just think, love-handle-free—and loving life.

The good news is, you're almost there. After the Single- and Double-Leg Stretch, add a Single Straight-Leg Stretch, Double Straight-Leg Stretch, and Crisscross. Don't forget that if your neck muscles give out before your belly, lower your head to the Mat or put one hand behind your head for support. Don't strain. To help establish a continuous tempo, focus on your breathing.

Even while pushing your powerhouse to the max, maintain butt-cheek tone. Now is a good time to introduce *push from the tush.* This push comes from a pinch in the lower tush, inner thigh, back of the thigh, and lower belly; it helps to safely lift your straight legs from the floor up to the ceiling. In other words, pinching your tush provides a little extra trunk support and tones your tush.

The movement and breathing patterns vary from exercise to exercise, so follow the pictures.

Perform the Single Straight-Leg Stretch in these steps:

1. You're on your back, and you've just finished the Double-Leg Stretch, with your knees into your chest.

2. Your chin on your chest lifts your shoulders off the Mat. At the same time, lift one leg to the ceiling, holding your ankle or calf with both your hands while extending the other leg to the side wall, about eye level. Now, pinch your butt cheeks.

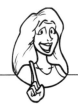

Pilates Lingo

As the difficulty of the exercises increases, you'll move with outmost muscle control. Whenever you read "push from the tush," initiate the movement from your bottom: your tush, your upper thighs, the back of your upper thighs, and your powerhouse.

3. Inhale and pulse the lifted leg twice. Exhale and switch your legs to pulse the other leg, keeping your legs straight the whole time. Imagine scissoring your legs to establish a rapid rhythm. Don't forget to blow out every ounce of air and make the belly as flat as possible.

4. Repeat 5 to 10 times, and then bring both your legs up to the ceiling to prepare for the Double Straight-Leg Stretch.

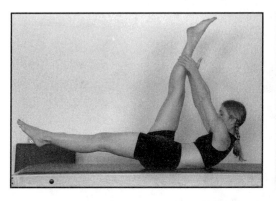 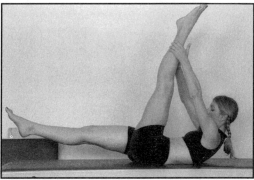

Perform the Double Straight-Leg Stretch in these steps:

1. As your toes lengthen out of your hip joints to the ceiling, clasp your hands behind your head for support.

2. Scoop your belly button in and up, and be heavy in your torso.

3. Inhale to lower your legs to the floor. Only take the legs as low as the back will allow: no strain, no arch, no bulge!

4. Exhale to lift your legs to the ceiling, blowing out every ounce of breath to make yourself skinny.

5. Push from the tush, meaning that the lift initiates from the lower tush, the inner thigh, the back of the thigh, and the lower belly—scoop in and up! Do 5 to 10 raises.

6. After you're done, pull your knees into your chest, but keep your shoulders up off the Mat so that you can transition into the Crisscross.

Pilates Precaution

If you have lower-back problems, skip the Double Straight-Leg Stretch. Or, if you feel that you'd like to try, bend your knees to reduce some of the pressure on your lower back. In addition, keep your toes pointing toward the ceiling; the higher your legs, the less stress on your back.

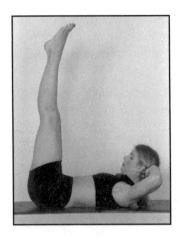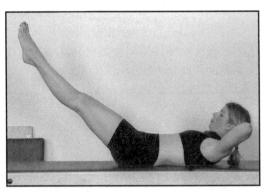

Perform the Crisscross by following these steps:

1. Extend one leg about eye level, while keeping the right knee toward the chest. Lift your chin to your chest.

2. Inhale and twist your torso, with your elbow reaching to the ceiling and your armpit to your knee. Twist a little farther each time as you count to three.

3. Exhale, and switch arms and legs. On the twist, reach as far back as you can, and keep both shoulders off the ground.

4. Repeat 5 to 10 times.

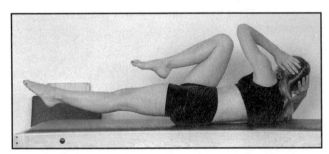

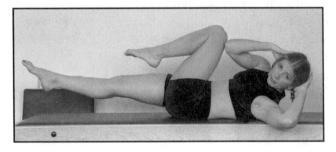

Double-Leg Kick

Got stress? Who doesn't? It will most likely affect how you hold your shoulders and upper back. The Double-Leg Kick, then, is a thorough stretch for your chest and upper back. It's also a total mental challenge because it tests your coordination skills. For example, your body moves in three different directions: Your head turns as heels draw into your bottom, while your arms shave up and down your back.

To modify this exercise, kick just the legs or do the arms only. In other words, divide the multiple movements into one. As you progress, then you can put them together.

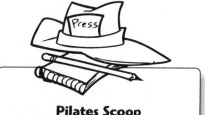

Pilates Scoop

Whenever you're on your belly, don't flab it. Scoop your navel to pull your abdominals to the spine and maximize your power-house.

After you perform the Single-Leg Kick, do the Double-Leg Kick immediately.

Steps to the Double-Leg Kick are these:

1. Lie on your stomach, with your right cheek on the Mat—don't let your belly button touch the Mat.
2. Clasp your left hand around two fingers on your right hand, and position them in the middle of your back, elbows to the floor. You should feel a nice stretch.
3. Inhale to cue your body.
4. Exhale and draw your heels to your bottom.
5. Pulse three times to get the hamstrings working. Be careful; don't lift your thigh bones off the Mat.
6. Inhale into extension, pinching your tush while shaving your arms down your back to lift your chest off the Mat. The shoulder blades should pull together to roll the shoulders back as you lift your clasped hands toward the ceiling to ensure a good chest stretch.
7. After that, you'll turn your head so that your other cheek touches the Mat.
8. Repeat the sequence four times.

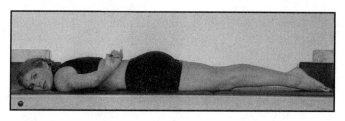

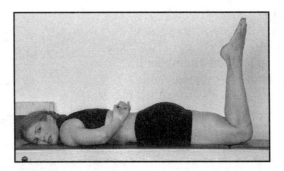

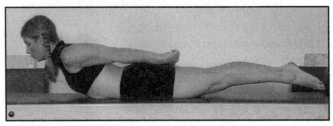

Shoulder Bridge (Stability)

Remember the 6–12 curl and imprinting the bones of the spine? The Shoulder Bridge is a perfect example of how the mini-exercises are built into the actual move. Plus, you'll fine-tune your bottom and hamstrings along the way. You're stretching your quadriceps, on the flip side, and the very tight back of neck muscles.

For now, you'll work on stabilizing your hips and keeping your spine in neutral as you build powerhouse strength. Your trunk should remain flat and rigid while your hips stay even and calm. The tendency is for the pelvis or one hip to sink. Imagine a yard stick balancing on your thigh bones.

To build your strength, you're going to extend your leg straight out. Hold for a count of five, and then place the leg down. But first just warm up the spine by peeling up and down. Read the directions for more details.

Build your Shoulder Bridge with these steps:

1. Lie on your back.
2. Place your feet about 8 inches apart as you anchor your entire foot to the Mat. Your elbows and shoulders are anchored as well as the back of head. Inhale to cue your body.
3. Exhale and start the pelvic curl, 6–12, to lift your spine off the Mat bone by bone. Count to five—1 Mississippi, 2 Mississippi, and so on. Inhale to imprint your spine, as if you're in the sand, to come down.
4. Repeat twice.

5. On the third time, lift one leg and hold it for a count of five. Return the leg, and readjust your hips to lift the other leg. You're striving to keep your hips even—no sags.

6. Repeat once. Imprint your spine, as if you're in the sand, to come down.

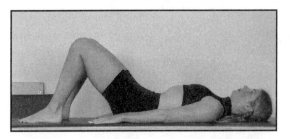

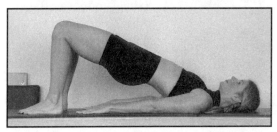

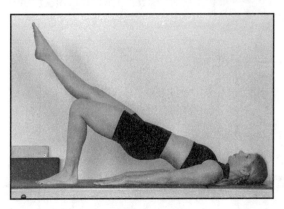

Teaser 1

C'mon, admit it, you're dying to test your stability and mobility while developing strength and flexibility. More than anything, though, the Teaser is a whole lot of fun. It's one of those exercises that tightens your tummy and jiggle-frees your behind. It's so true—your derriere gets a workout, too. All you have to do is tighten your tummy and push from the tush in harmony as you lift the body into a perfect "V" shape.

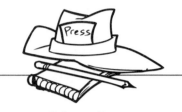

Pilates Scoop

The Teaser is a true test of your abdominal strength, and there are many variations of it. For example, place your feet on the wall about eye level. Inhale to lift scooping the whole way; in addition, practice pushing from your tush. Feel the upper back of your legs and inner thighs working to bring you up. As you exhale down, push your heels against the wall to activate your hamstrings and glutes. You don't want to plop down.

Don't sweat it. There are many variations to prepare you.

Test your Teaser with these steps:

1. Sit on the Mat and roll your pelvis into a 6–12 curl to balance.

2. Wrap your arms underneath your legs to lift your knees up, with your toes dangling just off the Mat. Keep your knees in the frame of your body.

3. Inhale the leg, with your toes reaching to the ceiling. Scoop and stay steady in your pelvis.

4. Exhale and lower the left leg. Repeat with the other side. Again, focus on scooping to help stabilize your pelvis.

5. Do three lifts for each leg.

6. Lift one leg up and then the other so that both legs reach to the ceiling. Use your arms to support your legs, but work on your scoop, to build strength and protect your back.

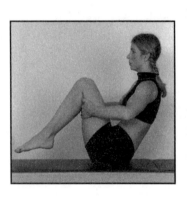 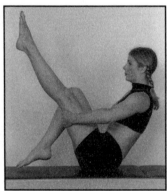 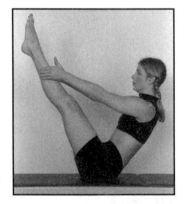

Let's Go Swimming

This exercise is the perfect coordination of upper- and lower-body strength, flexibility, and balance. You must stabilize not only in your pelvis, but in your shoulders as well. The tendency is for the hips to rock side to side as you lower and lift the limbs.

Think heavy in the torso, while scooping your belly button to the spine as your arms and legs move around your trunk. As always, draw your shoulder blades down your back to stabilize the shoulders!

As a prep, lift your right leg off the Mat and also your left arm. Your toes hover just a few inches off the Mat. Reach your fingertips to the side wall, while your toes lengthen out of your hips. Think yourself long as you fire the hamstrings, glutes, and lower-back muscles. Don't hunch your shoulders; stabilize by drawing your shoulder blades down your back. Hold for five counts, and then reverse limbs. After you feel comfortable with lowering and lifting your limbs, go for a swim.

Let's go Swimming with these steps:

1. Lie on your belly.

2. Lift your limbs off the Mat.

3. The rhythm is, inhale for five beats as you quickly alternate your arms and legs, lifting the torso a little.

4. Then exhale for five beats as you alternate your arms and legs, lowering the torso. Your pelvis is stable, and your head will come up, with the extension of the spine always following the line of the spine at all times.

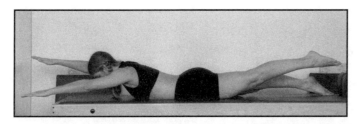

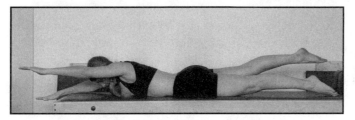

Head to Heel Like Steel: Leg Pulls

Here's your mantra: Head to heel like steel. Say it over and over again. These exercises challenge your total body strength: upper and lower body, plus core stability. Not only will you stabilize your pelvis, shoulders, squeeze your butt cheeks, and press your navel to the spine, but you also have to do this in midair. At this stage, you're developing enough strength to hold yourself up. Your head and toes will be in one straight line.

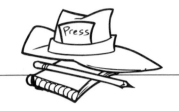

Pilates Scoop

Think: head, neck, spine, hips, legs in line the whole time when performing the Leg Pulls. The body remains in a straight line as your navel presses to your spine—no belly bulge.

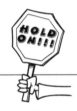

Pilates Precaution

If you have any wrist or shoulder problems, be careful with the Leg Pull Front and Leg Pull Back. If you have a wrist problem, you may want to work in a neutral wrist position, for example. If you have any pain, don't do the Leg Pulls.

However, there are rewards: firm butt, flat belly, sleek arms, while also stretching all the right places. Here's a warning: Depending on your strength or weakness, one hip may sink. Try to keep your hips even to challenge and not interrupt pelvis stability. Likewise, your belly must not sag in the Leg Pull Front. When you flip over to do the Leg Pull Back, on the other hand, you must not droop your fanny. You must stay head to heel like steel, in a straight line, to benefit from these exercises.

For a modified Leg Pull Front, get into the same position, but distribute your body weight on your elbow and toes. You can modify the Leg Pull Back the same way. Balance your body weight on your elbows and heels.

Strengthen the Leg Pull Front with these steps:

1. Lie face down on the Mat.

2. Press yourself up so that you're in a push-up position, with your arms directly under your shoulders.

3. Work to stabilize your hips, pull your navel to your spine, and pull your pits to your hips as you hold your body in a straight line. Also press your heels to the back wall, and keep your head to the front wall to work in opposition to keep the middle taut. Don't sag in your belly; imagine that a sharp needle is in line with your belly button. If you sag, then ouch! Stay lean and in a tight, straight line.

4. Repeat three to five times.

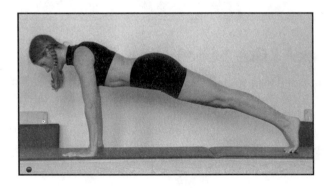

Develop the Leg Pull Back with these steps:

1. Flip over.

2. Place your arms shoulder width apart, with your fingertips either facing your heels or out to the side a little. Use the back of your legs to lift your bottom off the Mat, keeping your body weight traveling toward your heels.

3. Squeeze your butt cheeks, and reach your legs out of your hips to make a straight line from shoulders to toes. Don't let your tush sink. Think of a string pulling you up from your belly button, yet don't bulge your belly. Keep firm in your center.

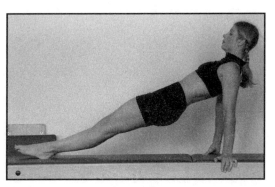

The Finish Line

Congratulations! You've just completed the six-week Mat workout, which covered basic and intermediate moves. These exercises will challenge you for some time. Stay here. Work on the moves to perfect your form. Focus on precision one week, then control another, and so forth. Remember, it's the details that make the move. Without details, moves are just moves. Why move through life, when you can flaunt it?

The Least You Need to Know

➤ Add the exercise Roll-Up as a transition into the next move so that the sequence of exercises keeps flowing.

➤ To increase the intensity of your workout, you must reduce the time, increase the difficulty of the moves, and challenge your muscles not to stop.

➤ Pilates trains your muscles so that they are prepared to live out everyday activities.

➤ Week 6 completes the shape-up basics, or beginner and intermediate work.

Part 3

Moving On Up

This part was written with two goals in mind: to challenge you and to provide work-outs for a lifetime. In the first two chapters, you'll learn the advance Mat exercises. As you get more efficient with the introductory work, you can turn to these chapters to challenge your body with moves that call for more strength, coordination, balance, flexibility, and control. As this part continues, you'll get the entire Side-Kick Series that will transform your legs and de-droop and de-dimple your bottom line. Finally, you'll learn to de-jiggle your arm waddle with exercises from the Standing Arms Series.

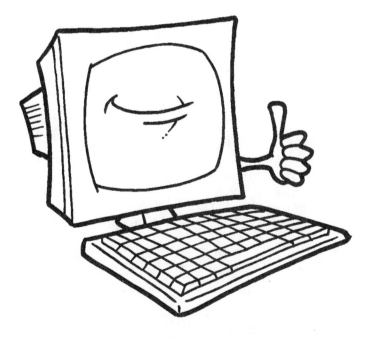

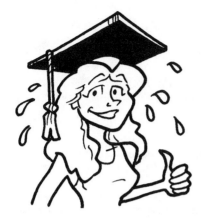

Chapter 9

Smart Sweating

In This Chapter

➤ Buff your dimples

➤ Putting an edge on the shape-up basics

➤ Theory of opposition

➤ Principle of self-resistance

Attention challenge-seekers: You're headed into the final stretch. Are you feeling stronger and more energetic, and even—dare I say it—breaking a sweat? No, not a pink-faced, dripping sweat; nevertheless, a little dewy under the arms and around your forehead.

A good sweat has many values. Besides detoxifying the body, it's a sign that you're working hard enough to condition the muscles, including the heart. A good sweat means that the intensity level is challenging enough to buff your body—even the dimples.

There's a great slogan: Buff your dimples! So, give up the antisweat dreams. In the end, a great body is really a matter of simple math—burn more calories than you take in. A little sweat is a sign that the caloric burn is heating up.

In this chapter, you'll add more intensity to some of the exercises that you've already done plus, learn a few new super-advanced moves, making the workout a bit harder. Yet you'll get the body you want and bask in a sense of accomplishment as you almost complete the sweaty Mat finish line.

Boosting Your Ability

Reach the head out of your neck as you lengthen your toes away from your waist. Sound suspicious? It's the subtle nuances that turn the internal furnace up to burn a few more calories. Think *theory of opposition*, which is a way to move your body in two different directions.

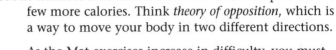

As the Mat exercises increase in difficulty, you must develop a certain awareness of how your body moves and muscles work. In other words, you're boosting your ability to fine-tune.

A Roll-Up works deep abdominal muscles—and that's probably where you felt most of the work, up to this point. When you work with opposition, not only will you use the muscles of the belly, but you also will use the hamstrings and inner thighs. You're learning to better control your movement and to activate as many muscle groups as possible.

As the moves increase in intensity, you must work in opposition. Let's take a closer look at the Roll-Up:

Pilates Lingo

The **theory of opposition** moves the body in two different directions to engage more muscle groups. It increases the resistance of all the exercises, and it gets you in touch with your body.

➤ **Opposition 1:** As you peel off the Mat, bone by bone, you'll press your heels out of your hips to activate the hamstrings. Your bottom is heavy, pulling down as the torso lifts upward. Stop here: Pushing the heels away from your hips counterbalances the weight of your trunk as it peels off the Mat. The deep abs are contracting, and so are the hamstrings as the body moves in a stable way. Hence, the body is moving in two different directions to control the move.

➤ **Opposition 2:** As you complete the Roll-Up, fingertips reach long past your toes, while the belly button pulls the abdominals back toward the spine. Translation: As your fingertips reach forward, so do your heels. The belly pulls back so that the body moves in two different directions—deep abs contract as the hamstrings stretch.

➤ **Opposition 3:** As the fingers reach past your toes, the pelvis moves into a 6–12 curl to continue to challenge the deep abs. And then you'll press the heels out of your hips to roll down bone by bone to engage the hamstrings; keep scooping. This weight in your bottom and heels gets the hamstrings contracting so that you have better control of the roll, and this prevents you from plopping down.

Control is crucial; it's safer, therefore, to work in opposition. If you roll down without pressing your heels away from your hips, here's what happens: Your hamstrings and inner thighs don't get a workout—or, worse, your legs may lift off the Mat, shattering your anchored position. You could get injured.

Tackling the Next Level

You've probably been doing just fine yet felt a little overwhelmed. After all, there are many exercises, breathing techniques, core concepts, and guiding principles to think about. By far, theory of opposition is a difficult concept to grasp. Nevertheless, incorporate it so that you get the most out of your workout: control, concentration, flow, and precision of movement.

Body awareness helps you move with control and precision. This resistance, in return, turns up the caloric burn. Being in touch with your body and how it moves while exercising is the best gift you can give yourself.

Before tackling the new moves, try the Mat exercises that you already know in opposition. I guarantee that you'll work that much harder. You'll find that you have more control and better form, and you'll ultimately engage more muscles. As you put this theory to the test, pay attention to the muscle groups that come into play. Of course, you'll reap all the usual benefits, but this extra challenge definitely tightens your look—precision, focus, and control never meant sweat-free.

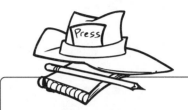

Pilates Scoop

Control is crucial! Working in opposition helps you control the moves a little better. Certainly, your focus will improve as you think about the two different ways to move your body.

What's Next?

Remeasure! Rejump! Don't step on the weight scale, though. Instead, your goal is to cut an inch, have fewer jiggles, or have extra room in your trousers. So take out the tape measure and evaluate the makeover progress. Be realistic, though. Don't expect a mega-reduction in inches; however, an inch is an impressive start.

Take this time to set new goals and write them down. You may want to take another set of pictures. You're shooting for another six weeks before remeasuring again.

There's no rush to add these exercises. They're super-advanced and are often done in an Advanced Mat class. The Mat work you've already learned can be done for months from now. Working in opposition will put a new spin on the movements.

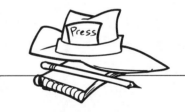

Pilates Scoop

Everything works in opposition: man, woman, sun, moon, winter, and summer. Our muscles, too, come in pairs that work in opposition; it's the key to life. When we work in opposition—with two ends working away—we keep the middle taut. If the legs relax, the middle sags; if the arms release energy, the middle sags, too.

In any event, the new exercises are as follows: the Rollover, the Jackknife, Spine Twist, and Push-Ups. And then there are the advanced versions to some moves that you've learned earlier: Swan Dive, Shoulder Bridge, Leg Pull Front and Back, and the Teaser. You're definitely not missing a muscle. Here's the entire sequence of exercises:

➤ The Hundred

➤ Roll-Up

➤ Rollover

➤ Leg Circles

➤ Rolling Like a Ball

➤ The Fives: Single-Leg Stretch, Double-Leg Stretch, Single Straight-Leg Stretch, Double Straight-Leg Stretch, and Crisscross

➤ Spine Stretch

➤ Open-Leg Rocker

➤ The Corkscrew 1

➤ The Saw

➤ Swan Dive

➤ Single-Leg Kick

➤ Double-Leg Kick

➤ Neck Pull

➤ The Bridge (kicks)

➤ Spine Twist

➤ The Jackknife

➤ Side-Kick Series (see Chapter 11, "Anticellulite Solution")

➤ Teaser 3

➤ Swimming

➤ Leg Pull Front (kicks)

➤ Leg Pull Back (kicks)

➤ The Seal

➤ Push-Ups

Control Is Crucial: The Rollover

This exercise tests your spine flexibility. It also works the deep abs and back muscles as you roll down bone by bone; you might even feel a little stretch in the hamstrings as you articulate the length of the spine. The Rollover tests your opposition. Picture this: As the legs go over the head, glue your abs to your spine the whole time—legs one way, abs the other.

Don't be surprised if you can't lift your hips over your head. Again, the Rollover requires a tremendous amount of belly strength. So, try this modification. Follow the same directions, but make a diamond with your legs. Inhale to lift your hips over your head; exhale to roll down bone by bone. Repeat three to five times. Do this prep until you get enough strength to lift the legs over your head, as seen in the pictures.

The movement is a little tricky. You'll start with the legs closed. Roll over and then open the legs to roll down. Reverse the leg sequence; open and close to roll down the spine as if a string of pearls is hitting the Mat one at a time.

Perform your Rollover with these steps:

1. Lie on your back with your hands by your side, palms down.

2. You have two options for your legs: lengthen your toes to the ceiling to anchor your tailbone to the Mat, which is slightly easy; or, for a super challenge, lengthen your toes out of your hips. However, you must have enough belly strength to keep your back anchored to the Mat at all times.

3. In one movement, inhale and push from the tush to lift your hips over your head, keeping the legs closed. Hover your toes a few inches off the Mat, keeping the knees directly over your eyes. Reach your fingertips long so that the weight of your body doesn't land on your neck. Notice the scoop!

4. Open your legs just past your shoulders. Exhale to roll down your spine bone by bone, and feel each bone as it lengthens the spine. Control the roll four ways: Press the back of your arms into the Mat, lengthen your toes away from the hips so that the weight of your bottom doesn't pull you down, reach your fingertips long as you roll down, and keep scooping.

5. When your tailbone touches the Mat either stop or swing the legs down to the Mat. If you take the legs to the Mat, keep your back anchored. If you can't, then just swing the legs until your back comes off the Mat. At that point, push from the tush and squeeze upper thighs to lift the legs back over the head, again.

6. Do three sets with the legs closed and then another three with the legs open, for a total of six.

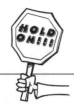

Pilates Precaution

If you have had any neck or upper-back problems leave this exercise out. In addition, if you have high blood pressure or a condition called macular degeneration, then you should not do any moves that put too much pressure on your head, the Rollover and the Jackknife, specifically.

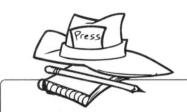

Pilates Scoop

All the exercises move in opposition. This is for three reasons: to add more resistance to the move so that the body works a little harder, to work the body with control, and to protect the body from injury. Moving in opposition takes the exercises to the next level—precision, control, focus!

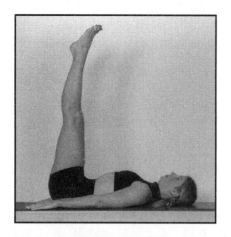

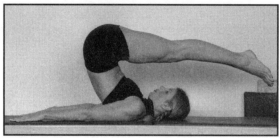

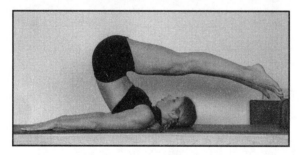

Hush Your Hips: Shoulder Bridge with Kicks

Now you're ready to add some kicks to the Shoulder Bridge, which, of course, cranks up the intensity. The goal is to kick and keep your trunk completely still. As Joseph Pilates said, "Quiet hips." When you kick the leg to the ceiling, the tendency is for the hips to sink—imagine that a sling hangs from the ceiling to hoist your hips to prevent your bottom from sinking into the Mat. Resist by pressing the foot of the standing leg into the Mat as if you're pushing your hips up as well. To refresh your memory, the Shoulder Bridge works all the right areas: the powerhouse, the glutes, the hamstrings, and the inner thighs.

Kick start your Shoulder Bridge with these steps:

1. Lie on your back. Your feet are about 8 inches apart as you anchor your entire foot to the Mat. Your elbows and shoulders are anchored as well as the back of your head. Start the 6–12 pelvic curl to lift your spine off the Mat—bone by bone. Stretch out a leg in front of you.

2. Inhale to kick it to the ceiling.

3. Exhale as the leg comes down, reaching the toes out of your hips. You can flex your foot for added bonus. Don't droop your bottom, and stay firm in your trunk.

4. Do three to five kicks with one leg, and then switch legs.

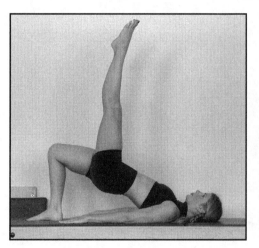 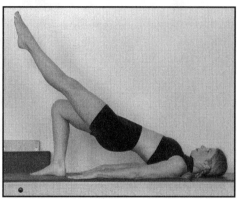

It's a Stretch: Spine Twist

Here's a treat! The Spine Twist is a breathing exercise to detoxify the bad air out of your body, plus it's a spine-soother. However, it's not as easy as it looks. As you rotate the spine, concentrate on cementing the body from the hips down. The tendency is for you to shift your hips as you twist—remain stable.

The "twist" is similar to the Saw. Lift up out of the hips, turn your belly button, and then twist. Remember, pinch, lift, and grow! Stay anchored from the base of your spine to the very top of your head. Finally, grow your fingertips long from your arms as you twist each time. That's how you'll get the delicious spine stretch.

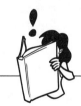

Pilates Primer

Your lungs are like a sponge. Squeeze the dirty water out to let the clean water in. In the Spine Twist, squeeze the dirty air out, and let the good air come in.

Soothe the spine with the Spine Twist in these steps:

1. Sit on the Mat, and pinch, lift, and grow! Legs extend long in front, with your heels and hips glued together and your feet flexed.

2. Think heavy in the tush, as if anchored down in cement from the hips on down. Arms extend out to the sides as you reach your fingertips long. Inhale to lift up out of your hips.

3. Turn your head to see your wrist, exhale, and twist, pulsing two times to ring the dirty air out of your lungs. Inhale to return to the center to exhale and twist the other way.

4. Do three to five sets.

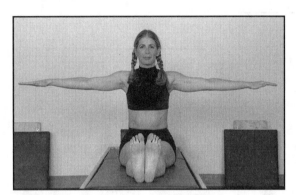 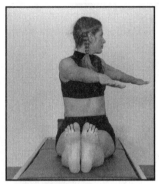

Straight as a Pencil: The Jackknife

Power up your powerhouse! The Jackknife is the ultimate test of powerhouse strength as you stretch the muscles in your neck, back, and shoulders. The Jackknife is similar to the Rollover; it challenges you to work bone by bone, only from a shoulder stand position.

The movement must be done with the outmost concentration, control, and flow. Imagine a constant flow with the legs—over the head, to the ceiling, and then down to the floor. Be careful: Don't jerk yourself up or let yourself plop down. Use your powerhouse to guide you down. The challenge is to keep your feet directly over your eyes as you roll down—now that's powerhouse strength.

Generate the Jackknife with these steps:

1. Lie flat, with your legs extended out in front of you on the Mat.

2. Press the back of your arms into the Mat, palms down.

3. In one flowing motion, inhale to lift your legs over your head, pushing from the tush and squeezing your butt cheeks and upper inner thighs. Think Saran Wrap!

4. Lift your hips up to the ceiling, pinching your butt cheeks, to a shoulder stand. Keep pinching so that you have that little extra lift. Pinch your butt, and the

pelvis pushes forward to lift you into almost a straight line from your shoulders to your toes.

5. Press the back of your arms into the Mat for support. Be careful—stop if you feel any pressure in your neck. Exhale as you roll down, keeping your toes directly over your eyes as you roll bone by bone; keep them reaching to the ceiling as if someone is holding your big toes!

6. Reach your fingers away from your shoulders for support, plus use your power-house.

7. Finish by lengthening your legs to the floor.

8. Repeat three to six times.

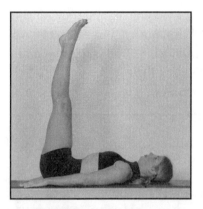

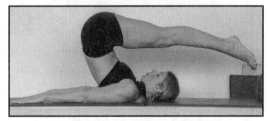

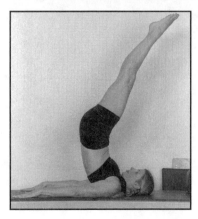

Just Not Any Only Old Teaser: Super-Advanced

Up to now, you've been practicing. Good, because you need powerhouse strength for the Advanced Teaser. If not, go back to the basics; otherwise, you may hurt your back. For example, you might throw yourself up, inadvertently straightening your back in the process, which may cause injury. Instead, push from your tush to help you up. Pinch your butt cheeks, and squeeze the backs of your upper thighs. Of course, power your powerhouse.

Test your Advanced Teaser with these steps:

1. Lie flat, with your legs extended out in front of you on the Mat. Press the back of your arms into the Mat, palms down.

2. Inhale to bring your arms and legs up simultaneously to make a "V"—fold yourself like a taco! Reach your fingertips to your toes.

3. Your trunk stays absolutely still as you lift your arms to your ears. Exhale to unfold the "V," scooping the whole way down to the Mat.

4. Repeat three to five times.

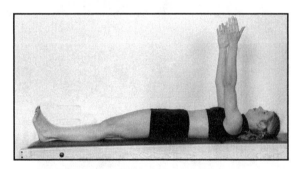

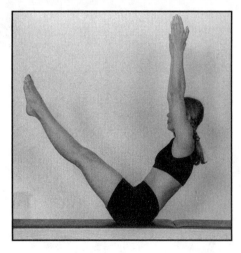

Head to Heel Like Steel: Leg Pulls and Push-Ups

Head to heel like steel, again! This time, you have kicks involved. After the stabilization work, you should have enough powerhouse strength to add a little extra oomph! Plus, you'll feel a nice stretch in the back of your calves.

Remember, you don't want to break your hips—keep them even and suspended.

Create the Leg Pull Front with these steps:

1. Lie face down on the Mat.

2. Press yourself up into a push-up position. Glue your abs to your spine—no belly flab! The palms of your hands are directly under your shoulders.

3. Press your shoulders down, pits to your hips. Stay lean and tight in a straight line.

4. Inhale to lift your leg to the ceiling while simultaneously rocking your other heel back and forth; it's a rhythmic motion on the ball of the foot.

5. Exhale to put your leg down. Keep your head in line with the spine the whole time. Don't sag the belly; imagine a needle in line with your belly button—ouch!

6. Repeat three sets of kicks.

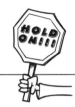

Pilates Precaution

If you have a wrist injury or a shoulder problem, skip these exercises. Or, you can try to work with the wrist in a neutral position, perhaps making a fist and performing these on your elbows. In any event, use caution with these exercises.

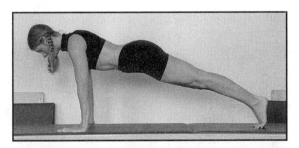

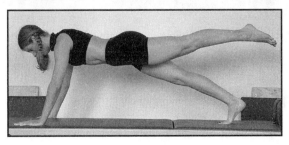

Going the Other Way: Leg Pull Back

Now stabilize the hips going the opposite way. This time, you'll kick the leg to the ceiling. As you kick up, stay firm in your center to stabilize your body. As the leg comes down, resist gravity and the weight of your leg by pushing your hips up. To get an additional stretch in the back of the leg, lead with your heel as you lower the foot.

Strengthen the Leg Pull Back with these steps:

1. Sit on your bottom.

Pilates Scoop

Flexing and pointing the foot are raisins on the cake. You can add these for extra challenge.

2. Place your arms a little wider than your shoulders, fingertips facing your butt or out to the side a little.

3. Lift your behind off the Mat. Squeeze your butt cheeks and lengthen your legs out of you to make a straight line from your shoulders to your toes. Press your heels into the Mat, and without any movement from the torso.

4. Inhale and kick your leg up to the ceiling.

5. Exhale to lower your leg. Inhale and kick again.

6. Repeat the kick three times, and then switch legs.

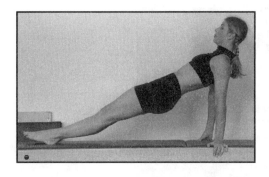
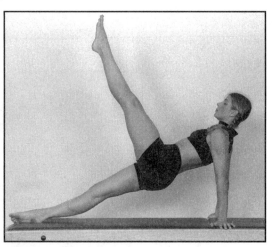

A Different Class of Push-Up

Everyone hates push-ups, but you won't hate this Push-Up! It's fun, and it tightens and tones just about every muscle. Of course, this Push-Up is a little different. You won't be missing a muscle: chest, shoulders, back, triceps, legs, and powerhouse while stretching. Engage the powerhouse fully; imagine a needle shooting through your belly button, if it sags.

If you can't get into proper Push-Up position, then you have two options: Do push-ups on the wall or on your hands and knees.

1. Stand up, feet in the Pilates "V."

2. Inhale and walk your hands down your legs in three counts, scooping the entire time.

3. Exhale to walk the hands out in three counts—still scooping—so that your palms are directly under your shoulders.

4. Remember, head to heel like steel as the crown of your head reaches long while the heels reach long in the other direction. (Notice a neutral fists position if you have a wrist problem.)

5. Inhale and bend your elbows, and lower your chest to the ground, shaving your elbows along your ribs. In other words, keep your elbows close to your sides.

6. Exhale to push up. Press your shoulders back and down as you push up to the head to heel like steel. Inhale as you walk your hands in. Exhale and hold the stretch while you scoop.

7. Then roll up, bone by bone, to a standing position.

8. Repeat three times.

And then look in the mirror, and say, "I've done a *wonderful* thing for my body." That's how you'll end your Mat workout.

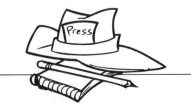

Pilates Scoop

The Push-Up is a perfect example of Joseph Pilates's brilliance. He took the traditional push-up, which primarily uses the chest muscles, and developed a Push-Up that calls for just about every muscle in the body while your legs still get a good stretch.

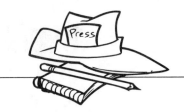

Pilates Scoop

For the super-advanced Push-Up, you can initiate the movement with one leg. It's the same steps, but you're balancing on only one leg as you go through the sequence. The tricky part is when you come up. You must use your powerhouse to balance your leg as you lift your torso up from the floor in one shift motion. Imagine a pendulum.

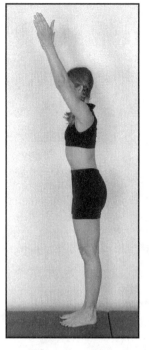
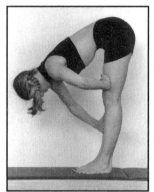
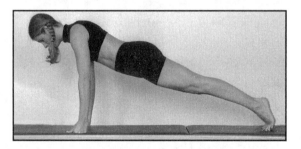
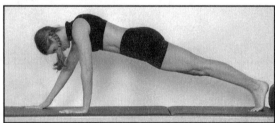
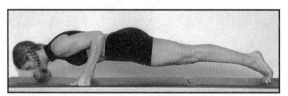

Be the Boss of Your Body

The goal: turn up the burn. Taking the Mat to the next level does this. You don't, however, have to add any more moves until you are good and ready. Remember, a move is just a move; anyone can memorize movements. The real work begins when you feel the exercise in your body and see it in your mind.

Be proud of your progress because you're teaching your body to obey your mind. Keep going—you're almost to the Mat finish line. And remember, scoop, length, squeeze, and pinch!

The Least You Need to Know

➤ A good sweat detoxifies your body and shows that you're working your muscles.

➤ Think *theory of opposition*—it's moving your body in two different ways.

➤ All the exercises work in opposition to increase the intensity, keep the movement safe, and control the movement.

➤ Joseph Pilates was a big fan of self-resistance.

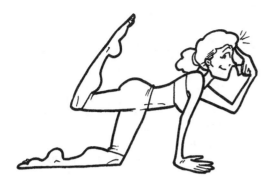

Chapter 10

The Intelligent Workout

> ### In this Chapter
> ➤ Use your breath to stop the mind from wandering
>
> ➤ Integrate your mind and body
>
> ➤ See it, and then do it
>
> ➤ Super-advanced moves to complete the series

You can't bend and twist your body into these moves without getting your brain involved. The Mat requires patience and uninterrupted concentration. It will challenge your physical limits, but it will bolster your will as well. The workout can be spiritual, holistic, and much more. Get in touch with that certain level of mind and body awareness that continues to propel you to the next level, and the next time, and then for a lifetime.

Body and Mind Integration

Distractions can destroy concentration. Yet it's your mind that creates most of the noise—at least, internal noise. However, you can learn how to turn off your thoughts and control your emotions with a mental training strategy called imagery. Elite athletes use imagery and visualization techniques to help them get ready for competition. So will you—not for competition, but to help you focus. After all, that's focus; it's clearing the mind so that no thoughts, emotions, or distractions take away from your ability to perform.

Ask yourself this: How do you see images? Close your eyes. Now imagine that you're doing a Roll-Up. Can you mentally describe the steps and how your body feels while going through the move? This will help you get your mind involved so that you take your workout to a higher level. You need to focus on whether you see, hear, or feel the movement; it's best if you can get as many senses involved as possible.

Do you experience the exercises from within, meaning seeing yourself performing them? Or do you see it through images? Both are equally important. Eventually you'll need to feel the exercises from within, even if you're not doing the moves. For now, you can rely on the images of these pictures to get you to that point. Try the following exercise to help your imagery.

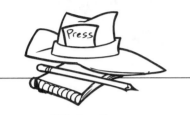

Pilates Scoop

To get your mind involved, you'll need to learn to create a mental picture of the exercise. Guided imagery is used to develop and execute the moves. Involve as many senses as possible so that you can create a vivid mental picture.

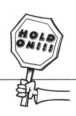

Pilates Precaution

As the intensity level of the Mat work increases, the mind will want to wander. Negative thoughts such as, "I look stupid doing this" or "I can't do this" seem to appear. Return to your breath to regain your concentration. Elite athletes must control negative thoughts, pregame jitters, and the emotional highs and lows of competition to perform well; it's done with imagery and breath control.

Sit in a quiet room or space. Close your eyes, and visualize the Roll-Up. Move slowly, smoothly, with full awareness and concentration moment to moment. If your mind wanders from the move—say, you're wondering what's for dinner—bring it back. Talk to yourself. Use verbal phrases and mental imagery to regain your focus. Repeat slowly in a monotone voice the core concepts. In your head, say "scoop" or "length" or "pinch." Focus on this word, and repeat it every time your mind wanders.

Give your mind vivid details: Scoop by gluing your abs to your spine. Feel this sensation by pulling your belly button in and up to the spine so that it's under your rib cage. The object is to use as many senses as possible so that the mental picture is complete. With that, the mind can better tell the body what to do.

For the next practice run, sit in a quiet room and watch yourself performing the Roll-Up, using your breaths this time. Notice how your muscles feel when you're breathing. If your mind wanders, bring it back with your breath. Smooth, rhythmic, harmonious breathing, along with mental tuning, helps you to develop a much higher level of concentration. One explanation may be that the center for breathing is located in a part of the brain where your body's lifelines are located: the controls for muscle tone, heart movement, blood circulation, and concentration. As we know, the breath can affect heart rate, blood pressure, and the nervous system. With fast, erratic breaths, your mind becomes scattered, while deep, rhythmic breaths can calm your mind.

You've probably noticed that when you intensely focus on something, you hold your breath. For example, as the intensity level of the Mat exercises increases, your mind gets fixed on one point, perhaps causing the mind to wander, making you think, "I can't do this move" or "I look so stupid." You're probably holding your breath as these negative thoughts float in and out. To erase negative thoughts, return to your breaths to keep you moving when you get stuck in negativity. Elite athletes must do this. It's vitally important to the outcome of their performance. They must learn to control negative thoughts, the pregame jitters, and emotional highs and lows of the event to perform well; it's done with imagery and breath control. You're no different. No, you won't be trying out for the Olympics, but you've got business deals and projects to conquer.

Practice makes perfect. Joseph Pilates designed each exercise with breaths so that you can work toward integrating your mind and body. Before each move, use imagery to cue your mind, and use the breaths to prepare your body. Do the exercise first in your head, and then move the body.

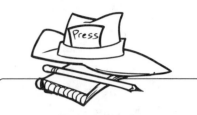

That doesn't preclude you from extra practice. You can practice imagery just before going to bed to refine your Mat technique, for example. Yet imagery and breath control are also useful strategies for everyday life. You can mentally prepare yourself to tackle a new work project or use breath control for those very stressful days. Still, we can all benefit from learning how to control the emotional highs and lows of life.

Pilates Scoop

Use your breath to move from within. By slow, rhythmic, and harmonious breathing, you can obtain a higher level of concentration and focus.

See It, and Then Do It!

Congratulations! You've entered super-advanced territory. Get ready to challenge your body to the max, yet it must engage your mind for help. Switch the focus from the actual move to moving in your mind. Use imagery and your breath to cue your mind and keep it focused as it wanders. Pay attention to how your body feels while setting up the move and how it feels while executing the move.

You can add these exercises when you feel ready. You don't have to tackle them all at once. For example, add the Scissors and the Bicycle only to your existing program. Still, you don't have to add these exercises at all, ever. You can stick to the basics for years to come and keep your body in great shape. There's always a way to challenge yourself a little more, something new to learn or a new way to feel it in your body and your mind.

Introducing the last eight moves: Swan Dive, the Scissors, the Bicycle, Hip Circles, Side Kneeling, the Mermaid, the Twist, and the Boomerang. Follow the sequence of exercises in order:

➤ The Hundred

➤ Roll-Up

➤ Rollover

➤ Leg Circles

➤ Rolling Like a Ball

➤ The Fives

➤ Spine Stretch

➤ Open-Leg Rocker

137

- ➤ Corkscrew 1
- ➤ The Saw
- ➤ Swan Dive
- ➤ Single-Leg Kick
- ➤ Double-Leg Kick
- ➤ Neck Pull
- ➤ The Scissors
- ➤ The Bicycle
- ➤ The Shoulder Bridge
- ➤ Spine Twist
- ➤ The Jackknife
- ➤ Side-Kick Series (see Chapter 11, "The Anticellulite Solution")

- ➤ Teaser 3
- ➤ Can-Can, Hip Circles
- ➤ Swimming
- ➤ Leg Pull Front
- ➤ Leg Pull Back
- ➤ Side Kneeling
- ➤ The Mermaid
- ➤ The Twist
- ➤ The Boomerang
- ➤ The Seal
- ➤ Push-Ups

The Swan Dive

Let's start with a Swan. Do two to three Swan preps to warm up the muscles in the back, and then try the Swan Dive. The directions are the same, but your arms don't touch the floor. The goal is to stay rigid in the body, keep the legs glued together, and lengthen the arms to the ceiling as you rock on the belly.

Visualize and feel your abs glued to your spine, which is especially important. Scooping protects the muscles along your spine; it doesn't take much to strain them—especially if you're rocking out of control. And pinch your butt cheeks, which also helps to control the rock. Remember: muscle, not momentum!

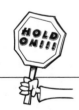

Pilates Precaution

Attention, men: The Swan Dive may cause a little discomfort to your privates as you rock. You may need to put a pad or pillow under your hips—perhaps near your thigh bones, or whatever is comfortable for you.

Rock the Swan Dive with these steps:

1. Lie on your stomach.
2. Place your hands directly under your shoulders, palms down. Elbows are glued to your rib cage.
3. Reach your toes long, as if a string is pulling your big toes.
4. Pinch your butt cheeks, scoop the navel to the spine, and press your shoulders back and down.
5. Inhale to straighten your arms to lift your head, neck, shoulders, and breastbone off the floor.
6. Exhale to lift your hands and drop your torso. As you rock, extend your arms out in front of you.

7. As you rock up, tighten your back as if the shoulder blades are drawing down your back, and lift from the back. Pinch as your legs go up, and scoop. Feel length in your body as you reach for a 10-carat diamond ring.

8. Repeat five times.

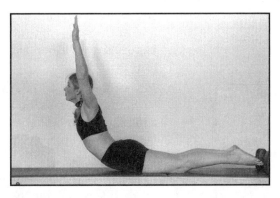

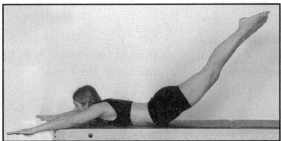

Age-Defying Moves: The Scissors and the Bicycle

Maintain quiet hips. Core stability is so important in these exercises; nothing moves but your legs.

Here's your first set of age-defying moves. The sequence starts with the Scissors and the Bicycle. The moves are rhythmic and nonstop, so you must correctly set the movement up before using your legs. Your powerhouse is to remain rigid in your trunk. Think about the opposition: Lengthen the leg to the side wall as the pelvis presses up to the ceiling.

Press your shoulders, elbows, and base of the skull into the floor for a solid base of support. As the legs move, the body presses up, defying gravity, as the legs go in opposition. Very little or no weight is placed on your wrists and elbows.

You've got to scoop and pinch your heart out to keep your body still as the legs move; it's a trial of core stability, strength and coordination. Plus, your bottom is getting a workout. If you want to try a modified version, turn to Chapter 16, "Spinal Soother: The Barrels." The Scissors and the Bicycle will be featured on the Low Barrel.

139

Split your Scissors with these steps:

1. Lie flat on your back with your arms out to the side, palms down.

2. Maintain core stability—legs long. Push your tush over your head, squeezing the backs of the upper thighs. Lead with your pelvis—keep pinching your butt cheeks so that your toes reach long to the ceiling. At the same time, place the palms of your hands on your lower back so that your bottom rests in your hands.

Pilates Primer

Joseph says: "Keep body rigid, move legs only .... Try gradually to execute 'split' so that toes of forward leg, in alternating movements, are beyond your vision; and backward leg, in alternating movements, likewise."

3. Anchor the back of the arm, from the elbow to your shoulder, to the Mat. Stay firm, scoop, and pinch your butt cheeks; it's this connection between your abs and glutes that stabilizes you as well.

4. In a split movement, inhale to lengthen one leg to the side wall while the other leg reaches past your head, pulsing two times.

5. Exhale to switch legs in a scissors-like motion, pulsing two times. After three sets of scissors, go right into the Bicycle.

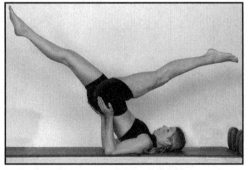

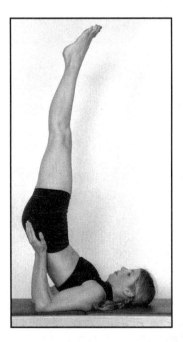

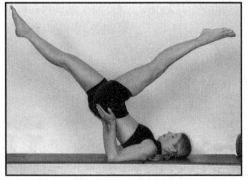

Put your feet on the pedals to cycle with these steps:

1. Inhale to reach the toes long to the side wall, down to your bottom and up to the ceiling, while lengthening your other leg to the ceiling.

2. Don't drop your knees into your face—lengthen, scoop, pinch, and stay firm. Imagine big cycles as you re-create the motion with your legs.

3. When your leg reaches the ceiling, exhale and start cycling the other leg. Repeat three cycles and then reverse the cycle.

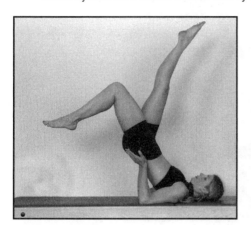 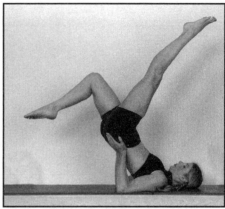

Let's Dance: Can-Can to Hip Circles

Get ready to Can-Can. After that, you can advance to Hip Circles. The focus is on deep abdominal strength, plus oh-so-much coordination. In the Can-Can, you're honing your coordination skills, which will come in handy as you progress to Hip Circles. If you have any back problems, don't progress to Hip Circles. The Can-Can is a safe and fun alternative. Eventually you can drop the Can-Can if you want. For example, after the Teaser, go right into Hip Circles.

Create the Can-Can with these steps:

1. Sit with your arms behind you, palms on the floor, or bend at the elbows.

2. Pull your knees into your chest, as close as possible. Point your toes and place them on a fixed point on the Mat. Elbows anchor to the Mat to prevent your trunk from moving and your shoulders from hunching. As you do the Can-Can, don't move your toes from that spot, and don't let your knees open.

3. Inhale to turn your knees to the right until you're sitting on the hip.

4. Still inhaling, bring your knees to the center, and then let them fall to the left; then quickly bring them back through the center to finish on the right side.

141

5. With the knees bent on the right side, exhale to reach the legs long to the ceiling, leading with your toes on the outside leg. Start left on the next sequence.

6. Repeat three to five times.

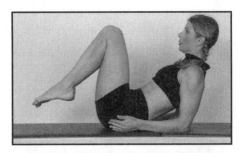

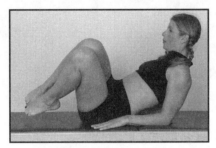

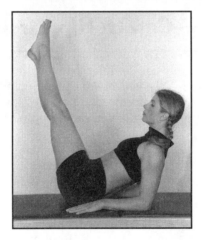

Hip Circles

When practicing Hip Circles, start small. The weight of your legs can pull your back into an arch. Be careful. You can also hold on to something (which is pictured) to help stabilize your torso. Your legs ultimately will reach out to the floor and then up, without arching your back. This takes a lot of powerhouse strength and lots of coordination.

Upgrade to Hip Circles with these steps:

1. Sit with your arms behind you, palms down, or hold something. Your arms stabilize your trunk, as does your powerhouse.

2. Bend your knees to your chest to lift your toes to the ceiling, and reach out of your hips.

3. Inhale to lower the legs to the left, down to the Mat—if possible, exhale to swing the legs up to the ceiling. Don't let your legs open—glue your ankles and knees together. You're drawing a circle on the wall in front of you; however, it doesn't have to be a big circle.

4. Reverse the direction.

5. Repeat three to five times.

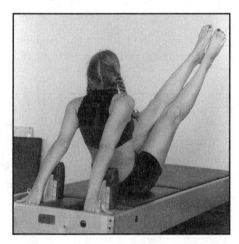 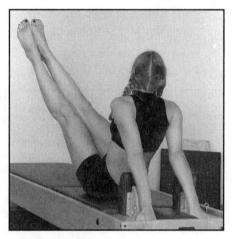

Precision Lifts: Kneeling Side Kicks, the Mermaid, and the Twist

This series is a long yet very beautiful set of moves. It starts with Leg Pull Back, which then transitions into Kneeling Side Kicks. After that, you'll stretch with the Mermaid. Then, you'll straighten your legs for the Twist. Whoa! You definitely have your fat-burning work cut out for you—but it's a lot of fun. The sequence flows to strengthen your bod!

Like all the exercises, these moves combine balance, strength, flexibility, and more strength. Yes, stretching, too.

Let's start with Kneeling Side Kicks. Focus on your waistline and hips. The goal is to stay firm in your core and let the legs do all the work. If you feel extremely wobbly, then don't kick. Just do the stability work and progress to kicking. In any event, start off with small kicks and make them bigger as your balance improves.

Perfect the Kneeling Side Kicks with these steps:

1. From the Leg Pull Back, bend your left knee while placing the palm of your hand into the Mat directly under your shoulder.

2. Push yourself up and lengthen your top leg out to the side.

3. Lift your leg so that it's in line with your hips.

4. Scoop to establish a good base of support between your knee and the palm of your hand.

5. Place your top hand behind your head so that the elbow points to the ceiling to open your chest and shoulders.

6. Inhale to kick to the front wall. Try to keep your leg at hip height.

7. Exhale to kick to the back wall, moving nothing except your leg. Don't sink your head and neck into your shoulders as you kick. Keep firm in the belly, and stay lifted in the waist.

8. After you complete four sets of kicks, drop your leg to the Mat, come back to the center, and do the other leg.

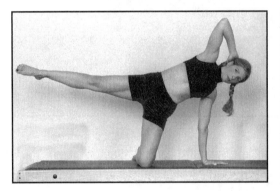 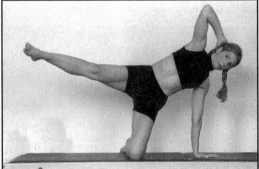

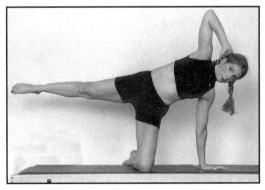

Pure Stretch: The Mermaid

Do the Mermaid with flowing arms and breaths. You're soothing the sides of your body with this stretch.

Stretch with the Mermaid with these steps:

1. Sit on the Mat.

2. Bend your knees and shift your weight so that your legs are underneath your derriere and you end up sitting on your left hip. Your right knee is on top of your left.

3. With grace, lift your left arm against your face in front of your ear to the ceiling, while your right hand stays on the Mat or holds your ankle.

4. Inhale to lift up and over your head to the right, stretching the left side. Exhale to center.

5. With one graceful motion, exhale to switch hands, and lift up and over to stretch the right side.

6. Repeat three times. And then switch legs.

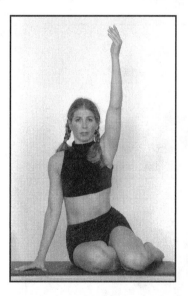 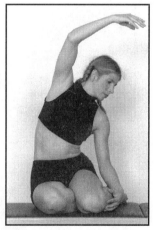

The Twist

The Twist is a pure power move that tests your balance and control. The goal is to stay absolutely still as you twist. If you can't, just lift and lower your body to build stability. Then progress to the actual Twist.

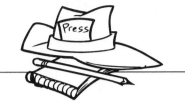

Pilates Scoop

Most of us push up and transfer all the weight to our wrist and shoulders. This is perfect opposition here. The arms and upper body work toward the feet, and the feet work toward the upper body to create a lift in the center so that we go up, not sink our body weight into our joints.

Test your Twist with these steps:

1. Sit on the Mat with your legs out to the side, and cross your top foot in front of your back foot.

2. Press the palm of your hand into the Mat while the other hand rests in front of your thighs. And scoop.

3. Inhale to lift your hips off the Mat, anchoring the palm of your hand directly under your shoulder while the other hand reaches over your head. The upper arm is by your ear as you look at the floor in a straight line from your toes to your fingertips.

4. Engage the muscles underneath your armpits to stabilize the shoulder and reduce the pressure in the supporting wrist and your body weight traveling toward your feet.

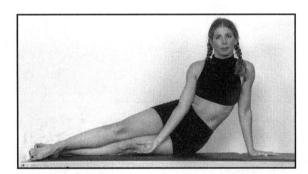

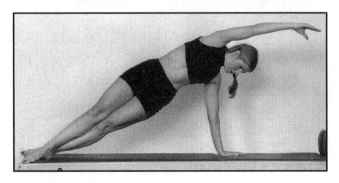

5. Remain firm as you exhale to lower your top hand as you sweep the floor, under your torso.

6. Inhale to twist back to open the chest while the top reaches back. Look up at the ceiling. The Twist is in the torso, not the legs. Imagine that your pelvis is the wheel that rotates the body around. Don't move or sink into your hips—stay firm. Exhale to lower the hips.

7. Repeat twice.

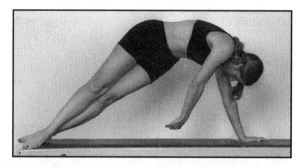

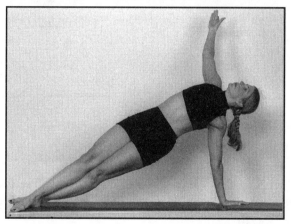

Balance in Motion: The Boomerang

Here's a story of a lovely lady who waits patiently for her prince charming. He shows up donning a beloved bow and arrow. After seeing this lovely lady, he imagines that her belly button is great for target practice. So, he fires and the arrow pierces the belly button, forcing the lady to scoop as she plunges back into the Boomerang.

The Boomerang is a perfect blend of balance, poise, strength, and flexibility; it works almost every muscle in your body. But you must scoop, scoop, and scoop to balance your body in motion.

Embrace the Boomerang with these steps:

1. Sit tall, with your legs straight in front of you.

2. Place your hands at your sides, palms down into the Mat. Cross your right ankle on top of your left ankle.

3. Inhale and, with the palms of your hands, lift up off the ground and go into a Rollover.

4. Lift your hips off the Mat so that your legs go over your head, balancing the weight on your shoulders, not your neck. Fingertips should reach long along the Mat.

5. Exhale to recross your legs quickly; the right ankle uncrosses so that the left ankle crosses on top of the right.

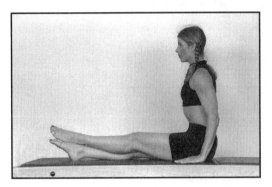
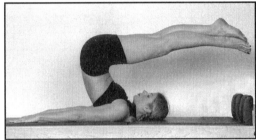

6. Inhale to slide the palms of your hands along the Mat to lift you into a Teaser, or "V" position. Scoop, scoop, scoop.

7. Exhale slowly as you balance, circle the arms down by your sides to lower part of your back, clasping your fingers and reaching your hands away from your body. Don't lose your scoop. Stay as still as possible while opening your chest to feel a slight stretch.

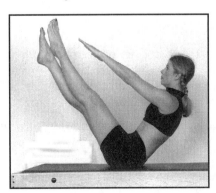
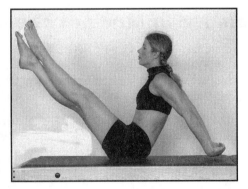

148

8. Raise your clasped hands up to the ceiling while slowly lowering your legs to the floor with absolute control. No plopping!

9. Unclasp your fingers, and circle the arms in front, reaching to the toes. Keep scooping, even as you stretch. The left leg is now on top and ready to boomerang again.

10. After two complete sets, you're ready to bark like a Seal ....

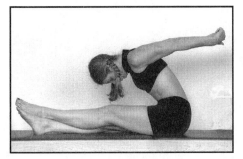 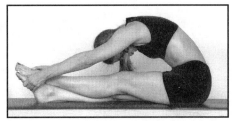

Last Call

Congratulations! This chapter completes the Mat exercises. As you've seen, the Mat requires a lot of practice, as well as focus, concentration, and precision. Remember, the Mat is just part of Joseph Pilates's methods. There are the machines, too.

This journey is just the beginning to help you get in touch with your body and mind. In this case, practice makes perfect. After a few months, you'll feel more confident, have less flab, and double your core strength. Be proud, because your total look will only get better as you continue to reshape from within.

The Least You Need to Know

➤ Breathing helps you concentrate and focus.

➤ Imagery is seeing the exercise in your mind.

➤ If you can see it, your body will do it.

➤ Don't do these exercises if you have wrist problems: Leg Pull Front, Leg Pull Back, Kneeling Side Kick, Twist.

➤ Every move is a delicate mix of balance, control, flexibility, and strength.

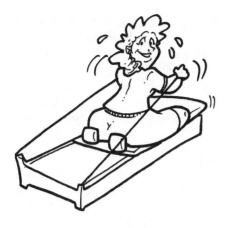

Chapter 11

The Anticellulite Solution

In This Chapter

➤ The anticellulite solution

➤ Legs to die for

➤ Firm up your bottom

➤ Still working the powerhouse

Does your butt have too much wiggle? Or a droop in need of a bottom lift? Do your legs jiggle like Jell-O? Does the popular television jingle "Watch it jiggle, see it wiggle …" come to mind as you walk? If so, then it's time to de-dimple and de-droop your derriere. No, a random dimple won't kill you, but those dimples should be reserved for our face cheeks!

You can tighten those areas that seem to outlast the Energizer bunny with the Side-Kick Series. Imagine a crusade against the unmanageable dimple—you won't ever have to feel defeated by the battle of dimples and saddlebags. This chapter is the anticellulite solution so that you can reshape your backside for good.

De-Fat Your Dimples

To sculpt the bottom half, you need to target the muscles that betrayed you—the muscles that got soft! The Side-Kick Series targets the muscles in your legs and derriere, plus the powerhouse; it's the powerhouse that stabilizes the torso so that you can move the legs.

All along you've been pinching your butt cheeks, lifting through the backs of your upper thighs, and scooping your transverse to the spine. Don't stop. The core

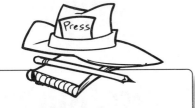

Pilates Scoop

How many words can you come up with to describe your buttocks? There's *patootie, butt, butt cheeks, derriere, heinie, behind, posterior, glutes, rear end, fanny, cheeky, backside, maximus, tail, rump, bottom, tush,* and *tuckus!*

concepts still apply here. It's these muscles—the pelvic floor muscles, the inner thighs, the hamstrings, and the lower abs—that help stabilize your pelvis as your legs move. Still, you sculpt many of the muscles that you are probably already familiar with: the quadriceps, which run down the thigh; and the hamstrings, traveling from your buttocks to the back of the knee.

Then there are smaller but not forgotten muscles: the *gluteus medius* and *minimus.* These muscles are strategically located on the outside of your thigh to work in harmony with the *gluteus maximus.* Slide your hand down the inside of your thigh. This group of muscles is called the hip adductors, while the muscles that run down the outside part of your leg are hip abductors, a.k.a. saddlebags.

Empowering Your Patootie

You'll start the legs off easy. In weeks 1 and 2, you'll do three exercises: the Side Kick, the Beat-Beat, and the Passé. As the weeks continue, the degree of difficulty will increase. In weeks 3 and 4, you'll challenge the core even more and work the leg muscles with more exercises that use larger range of motion. And then in the last two weeks, you'll add the most advanced moves to engage even more muscle fibers. Translation: tighter results.

Follow the captions that accompany these movements because they will tell you when to add these exercises to your existing Mat routine. Remember, you're laying in exercises as the weeks go on. The Mat exercise Teaser will always follow the Side-Kick Series.

Don't stop between leg exercises. The Side-Kick Series was designed to rap-tap-tap along at a rhythmic pace. The series was brilliantly masterminded to gradually increase the workload so that you can transform the stubborn dimples. The Side-Kick Series is as follows:

- ➤ Side Kick
- ➤ Beat, Beat Up
- ➤ Passé
- ➤ Circles, Front and Back
- ➤ Parallel Leg
- ➤ Double-Leg Lift
- ➤ Close the Hatch

- ➤ Big Circles
- ➤ Flutter Kicks (small, medium, big)
- ➤ Hot Potato
- ➤ Grand Ronde de Jambe
- ➤ Bicycle (transition)
- ➤ Beats on the Belly (transition)

Stay Square

To de-dimple this area, you need to focus on the pinch and scoop in conjunction to work the legs and derriere. In other words, don't flab your tummy; it can't hang over your waistband.

The body position for the Side-Kick Series stays the same as you work from move to move. Here's the important part: Keep your hips stacked on top of each other, and stay square. The feeling is that the top leg is slightly heavier than the bottom, so the upper inner thighs shave past one another. Your knees slightly turn out as if you were in the Pilates "V." For example, turn your knee slightly to face the ceiling, leading from the hip joint while the bottom knee turns down slightly to face the floor.

Square off the shoulders as well. At first, you may feel wobbly as you kick, circle, and bend the leg. Staying square in the upper body as well helps to stabilize your torso. Keep in mind that when you're working the legs, the trunk must remain still. You can use your hand for additional support. You'll start in the beginner/intermediate position. If you have a neck or shoulder injury, then lower your bottom hand to the floor so that you can rest your head. You can also put a small pad between the support hand and your head, or whatever feels comfortable; it's important that you don't strain your neck.

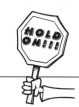

Pilates Precaution

The most common mistake is that students forget to press the palm of the top hand into the Mat, so the trunk wobbles and teeters as the leg swings back and forth, throwing off body alignment. In the end, they work the muscles incorrectly, work into the joints, or create muscle imbalances. Use the palm of the top hand like a bicycle uses a kickstand for support.

Strike a pose with this picture:

1. Lie in a straight line, with your neck, shoulder, hips, and legs in line.

2. Use your arm on the Mat to support your head, specifically the palm of your hand. The top hand acts like a kickstand; it provides support as the leg moves.

3. Press the palm of your hand into the Mat, and activate the triceps to help stabilize you along with your powerhouse.

4. After you're in position, lift your legs to the front of the body, about a 45° angle. The bottom leg reaches long, leading with the toes; turn them under. The top foot is in a soft point.

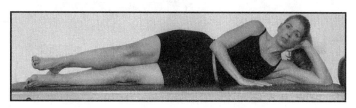

Off to Get a Better Butt: Weeks 1 and 2

In weeks 1 and 2, you'll perform three exercises: Side Kicks, Beat-Beat Up, Side Passé. And, of course, the Mat wouldn't be a workout if you didn't flow with a transition, so Beats on the Belly it is. Think Dorothy in *The Wizard of Oz*. She wanted to go home so badly that she clicked her heels together. Instead of seeing the wizard, you're off to get a tighter tush. So click, click, click.

Be careful: You may shock muscles that have been comatose. If you feel any burn or pain, do one more and then stop. No need to push yourself into a burn—less is always best. Don't forget to complete the Side-Kick Series on the other leg.

Here's the rundown on the working muscles: The Side Kicks work the inner and outer thighs, plus gradually warm the hip joints for more work to come. For example, Beat-Beat Up is a killer for the inner thighs; it stretches and flexes, yet doesn't neglect the hips and the butt. And then finish with the Passé; it, too, works all the right places: hips, inner thighs, and butt.

Let's start with the Side Kicks in these steps:

1. Get in position. Lift the top leg to hip height, and slightly turn up the knee leading from the hip joint.

2. Inhale and, with your hips stacked, swing your leg forward, and then pulse two times. The rhythm is kick, and then another small kick. A common mistake is to roll your hips forward as the leg swings, but keep your hips stacked.

3. Exhale to swing the leg back, adding a small kick. Feel your bottom work, especially as you pulse on the second small kick. Watch out—your back may arch and your ribs may flare out as the weight of your leg swings back. Keep your ribs down and your hips stacked. After six to eight sets, put your heels together, as if kissing.

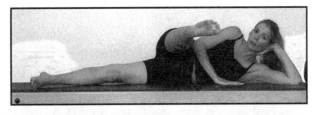

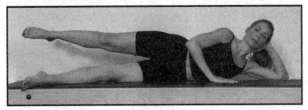

Follow up with Beat-Beat Up in these steps:

1. Inhale and lift the leg up to the ceiling; the knee leads the way. (You can add the beats later, if you want.)

2. Exhale to lower the top heel to the bottom heel, and pulse the heel quickly in front of the foot resting on the Mat and in back. Add some self-resistance as you lower to beat-beat. Here's the rhythm: beat-beat—UP! beat-beat—UP! Repeat this six times, and then seal it with a kiss—heels together.

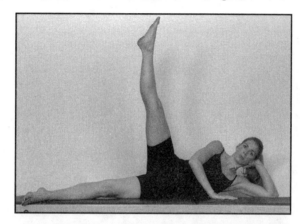

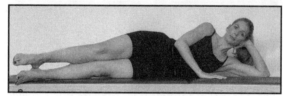

No pausing—go into Side Passé in these steps:

1. Inhale and slide the heel along the inside of the bottom leg, exposing your inner thigh the whole time.

2. Keep inhaling as you bend the knee and lengthen the leg to the ceiling.

3. Exhale and press the top heel to the bottom heel, saying, "One, two, three miles longer …." The top leg comes down longer than the bottom heel to create length.

4. Repeat three times, and then reverse the direction of the Passé.

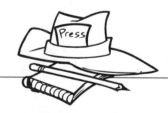

Pilates Scoop

The most important thing about the Side-Kick Series is to keep the upper body completely still as the leg kicks, circles, and bends. To do this, you must scoop, pinch, and stay square in the hips and shoulders.

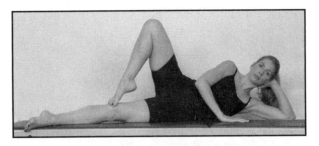

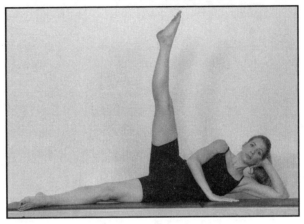

Finish with Beats on the Belly in this steps:

1. As gracefully as possible, roll onto your belly for Beats on the Belly.

2. Rest your head on your forearms in front of your head. Lift your belly button to your spine. Put a thousand-dollar bill between butt cheeks. Lift the legs off the Mat, about 2 to 3 inches.

3. Inhale to beat your heels together, counting to five.

4. Exhale while still beating the heels for another set of five.

5. Take a few seconds to rest in Child's Pose. Then complete these exercises on the other leg.

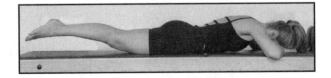

Bye, Bye, Butt Rut: Weeks 3 and 4

Let's target the hot spots: the patootie, the thighs, and the inner thighs. In these weeks, you'll add more leg moves that challenge the core even more and increase in range of motion. The Side-Kick Series gets harder and longer. Pay attention to how your body feels. Push it, but don't overdo it.

Focus on keeping your hips stacked. Watch for sloppiness. As the moves increase in difficulty, your body might sacrifice good form for bad form: sinking into your waist, lowering your shoulders, twisting your torso, or just working the leg incorrectly. Sloppiness always coexists with fatigue. Don't complete the set if you can't stay aligned.

Remember, the leg work is rhythmic—no stopping. In these weeks, you'll add Small Circles, Parallel Legs, Double-Leg Lift, Close the Hatch, Big Inner Thigh Circles, and Flutter Kicks. The transition is the same, Beats on the Belly.

Start with the Small Circles, front and back, in these steps:

1. From the Side Passé, lengthen the leg to the top heel as if it is working beyond the other heel, pulling from the waistline, knee facing up.

2. Lift the leg just about an inch. Keep the circles small so that the inner thighs shave one another.

3. Circle the leg five times, touching your heel with every circle. Work from the inner thigh down. In fact, try to touch the thighs—let no light in, so pinch your butt cheeks.

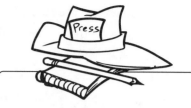

Pilates Scoop

In every exercise, you're strengthening and lengthening while developing coordination and control.

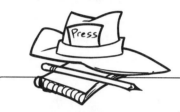

Pilates Scoop

Stay lifted from the top of your head to the top of the big toe. Think tall—6 feet tall to create length. Don't sink into your waist, lean back into your hips, or round your shoulders as you bend or kick. Stay square so that your legs get the workout they deserve.

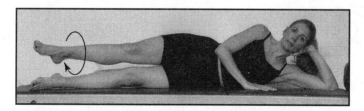

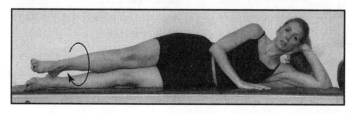

4. Reverse the circles for another 5, totaling 10 small circles.

5. Move the top leg so that it reaches back, keep the hips square. Circle 5 times, and then reverse for 5, totaling 10 small circles. Breathe normally. The leg stays back.

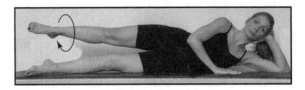

Next up, Parallel Leg. Follow these steps:

1. Flex the foot to work the leg in parallel. Make sure that the hips are stacked.

2. Inhale to lift the leg in three counts—a little higher each time.

3. Exhale to lower the leg in a one-count, as if the elevator just fell to the floor, squeezing the inner thighs.

4. Repeat four times.

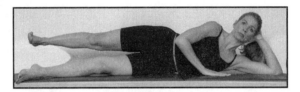

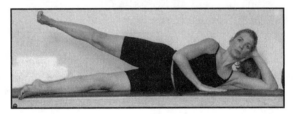

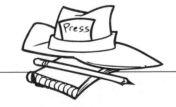

Pilates Scoop

To get the most stretch possible, lengthen your legs away from your waist when they're straight—imagine your legs starting from your belly button.

And then do Double-Leg Lift, using these steps:

1. Lower your head to the floor to rest on your arm.

2. Straighten the legs so that your body is in one straight line from head to toe.

3. Inhale to lift your legs off the Mat, keeping the knees and ankles together so that no light shines through.

4. Exhale to lower the legs. Repeat four times. On the fourth lift, drop the bottom straight leg to continue with Close the Hatch.

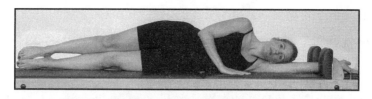

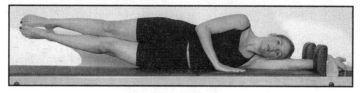

Follow up with Close the Hatch in these steps:

1. With split legs ...

2. ... Close the Hatch by lifting and lowering the bottom leg to the top leg.

3. Lead from the inner thigh on down. Breathe normally. Repeat five times, and then add Big Circles.

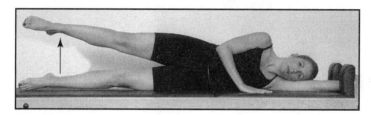

And do Inner Thigh Circles in these steps:

1. With split legs, the bottom leg circles, leading from the inner thigh, touching the heel every time. The rhythm is this: Circle 1, touch heel. Circle two, touch heel.

2. Repeat three circles, and then reverse the circle for three more, totaling six. Breathe normally. Then lower the legs to just about an inch off the Mat for Flutter Kicks.

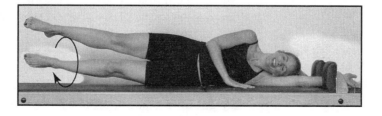

Put on the finishing touches with Flutter Kicks in these steps:

1. Squeeze your butt cheeks, and press the palm of your hand into the Mat to stabilize your torso. Nothing moves but your legs; it's a great butt move! Breathe normally.

2. Scissor your legs, making the scissors bigger and bigger.

3. Do about 10 flutters. Then you're ready to roll on your belly for Beats on the Belly.

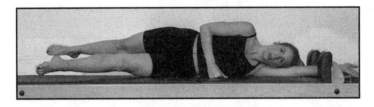

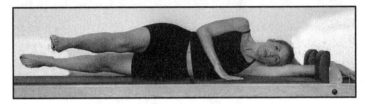

Giving Up Your Rear: Weeks 5 and 6

Worried about your butt? Don't. It's covered with these exercises, *Grande Ronde de Jambe* and Hot Potato. These moves are the quickest way to redefine your bottom because the exercises require big leg movements and powerhouse power. You're working to stabilize your torso as the movements in your legs get big, bigger, and biggest.

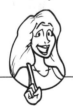

Pilates Lingo

In French, **Grande Ronde de Jambe** actually means "big leg circles." In fact, *Grande Ronde* translates to "big circle"; *de Jambe* means "of the leg."

Grande Ronde de Jambe translates to "big leg circles" in French. Hot Potato, my favorite, will definitely wake up your duff. Pay attention because you may find that the big movements are throwing off your base of support.

This exercise completes the Side-Kick Series. As you've been doing, follow the leg work sequence in order, one right after the other. There's one exception: You can replace Beats on the Belly for a new transition, the Bicycle. It's a complete leg stretch: quadriceps, hamstrings, lower back, and all the maximuses.

Here's the rhythm: After Flutter Kick, you'll be in a straight line. Reposition the legs to a 45° angle to complete Hot Potato and Grande Ronde de Jambe.

Then you'll finish with a thorough leg and hip stretch with the Bicycle. After the Bicycle, do the Russian Splits just for fun!

Do the Hot Potato in these steps:

1. Imagine that your big toe is touching a hot grill. You won't stay there long, so as the toe taps, lift the heel to the ceiling, staying square in the hips. Easy enough—don't forget to breathe normally.
2. Tap your big toe five times, in front.
3. On the fifth leg lift, the toe taps behind the supporting leg, near the heel of the bottom foot.
4. Lift and lower five more taps to the back. On the fifth lift, the toe taps front.
5. Tap three more and then behind for three more. Here's the hot, hot, hot part: On the third set, tap front, lift up, pause and then tap back, lift up, and pause only one time. The Hot Potato order: 5-5, 3-3, 1-1.

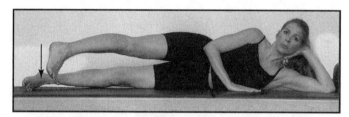

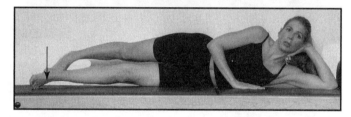

Challenge the thighs with Grande Ronde de Jambe in these steps:

1. Lift the top leg so that it's at hip height.
2. Swing your leg to the front wall. Look at your knee.
3. Watch your knee as your leg circles to the ceiling. Here's your tip: As your leg circles front and up, keep your knee up the whole time!
4. Rotate the leg to the back wall so that your knee is in line with your belly button. This rotation comes from your hip socket. Be careful: The weight of your leg may pull the hips back. Stay square, and press that top hip into the bottom hip as the leg swings.
5. Your leg swings down to finish the circle, sweeping past the heels to keep the flow.

6. Circle three times, breathing normally. Then reverse the pattern: Swing your leg back up, to turn in the hip socket and around to the front, pressing the hips square to counterbalance the weight of the leg.

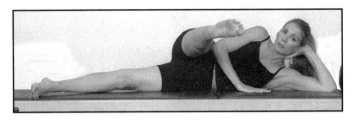

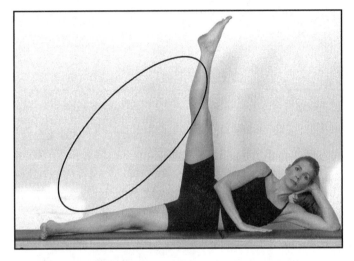

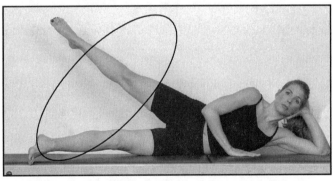

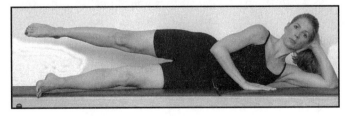

Finish with the Bicycle in these steps:

1. Lift your top arm out by your head, and hold it there.
2. Kick the top leg to your arm.
3. Bend your knee and bring it into your chest, as if to kiss your knee.
4. With your knee bent, bring it back so that your heel touches your belly button. Don't lift any higher than the hip.
5. Reach the bent knee to the back while reaching your top arm long, stretching from the fingertips to your toes.
6. Repeat the cycle three times, and then reverse it. Keep the movement slow so that you feel each stretch. Breathe normally.

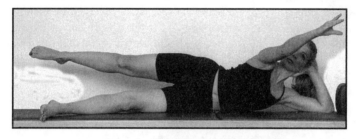

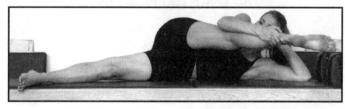

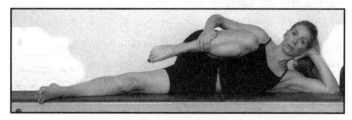

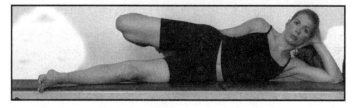

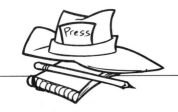

Pilates Scoop

The big leg circles are a challenge for many students. The most common mistakes are the hips sinking and the waist collapsing as the leg circles. Resist this urge by pulling out of your head and waist, and keeping your ribs in.

After six cycles, you can do the Russian Splits. Then continue the Side-Kick Series on the other leg. Then it's time for the Teaser.

Boosting Your Bottom Line

Can you alter your backside? After all, the shape of your patootie was chosen long before you donned a diaper; it's called heredity. No matter what your God-given right, you can shift what you were born with. A healthful diet and these moves can make the most of what you've got. Your goal is to pass the "I can't hold a pencil between my butt cheeks and leg crease" test. In other words, be proud that the pencil drops to the floor. You're on your way to boosting your patootie, derriere, fanny, or my grandmother's favorite—tuckus!

The Least You Need to Know

➤ Muscle takes up less space than fat. As you develop muscle, you'll get more compact, thus reshaping your backside for good.

➤ The Side-Kick Series is made up of 11 exercises that de-dimple your button and shrink your saddlebags.

➤ The important part: Keep your hips stacked on top of each other, and stay square during all the leg work so that you don't work the wrong muscles.

➤ Stay lifted from the top of your head to the top of the big toe. Think tall—6 feet tall, to create length. Don't sink into your waist or lean back into your hips, and don't round your shoulders.

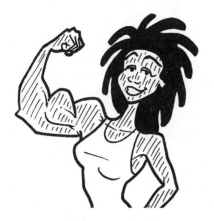

Chapter 12

Flexing Muscles

In This Chapter

➤ All about stiff necks

➤ Tension tamers

➤ Upper body, belly, and leg exercises

Whittle away your waddle. You know, the flabby skin that waddles long after you've lifted your arm to, let's say, wave good-bye—it just keeps jiggling and jiggling …. You can have the arms you so deserve. These exercises roll into one: sleek arms, strong back, flat abs, and lean legs. How? While toning your arms, you'll still focus on your powerhouse and legs.

Not only will you look good, but well-toned arms also can protect you from upper-body strain, including your back and neck. You'll lift heavy shopping packages, you'll twist to hoist your child from the floor, and you'll sit hunched at a computer all day multitasking—type, talk, and, twist.

What makes lifting, typing, and twisting a breeze? Toned, jiggy-free arms. The good news is that arms respond to exercise super-fast. Why? Because the muscle groups in the arms are smaller than your thighs—and, for most of us, there's less fat that wobbles. So, you'll see results fairly quickly.

Dust off your dumbbells, because you're about to use them to super-sculpt your arms and upper back. These exercises target all the right muscles: deltoids, rhomboids, latissimus, trapezius, biceps, triceps, and not to mention the smaller muscle groups that enhance your posture. So get ready to get jiggy-free!

To Tense or Not to Tense

What's the long-term result of overtensing the muscles? Dysfunctional muscles. Here's why: a buildup of lactic acid in the muscle fibers. Lactic acid, we know, is a waste product of working muscles, which dissipates as the muscle rests. However, let's say that your muscles are always tense—turned on and overworked.

Then the problem is two-fold. When muscles are always working, you can usually feel the effects before the results. You might be sore and stiff, in other words. However, there's a silent enemy within. If your muscles don't relax—let's say, because you're constantly tensed—then lactic acid also builds.

Whatever the case, an accumulation of lactic acid can cause injury to the tissue. Injuries to the muscles can compromise the way it responds. For example, a muscle might not be able to reach its normal length; it has shortened, and so has your movement. Is this a problem? You bet. The body is a closed system, lining up from the head, neck, shoulders, hips, knees, and feet. If one part is misaligned, then that means trouble for the rest of your body. The body will do anything to work as naturally as possible, even if that means sacrificing other muscle groups to compensate. Constriction throws off the natural rhythm of your body.

We hold most of our tension in the neck, shoulders, and upper back. The upper trapezius (or traps, for short), then, is the most overused muscle. Not only do we tense up for the day-to-day stress, but we also spend most of the day hunched over a desk or lifting heavy objects. As the upper trapezius overworks, the lower traps are underused; weak arms compound the problem. After all, if you don't have the arm strength, then either your neck or your back will pick up the slack. Translation: An overused upper back results in an aching back.

If you can recognize and let go of tension in the upper traps, then you're working toward releasing it. You can save a lot of wasted energy, which can be put to better use. Many of these exercises can help, too. Think about keeping your shoulders back and down; hang your shoulders, and keep your pits to your hips to unglue your shoulders from your ears. Besides reinforcing good body alignment, you're not creating any extra stress in the upper back, which needs no extra stress.

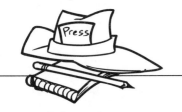

Pilates Scoop

Combat the stress and get it out of your body—just by telling it to go! Lift your shoulders to your ears and then release so that they are heavy. Soften your neck and relax your jaw to take the stress out.

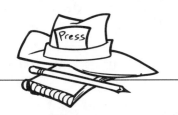

Pilates Scoop

The most overused muscle in your body is your upper trapezius. Not only does it hold tension for the day-to-day activities, but it also compensates for weak upper body strength.

My Stiff Neck

So you're desk-bound and your neck aches. How are you holding your head. Does it hang forward? Overworked, overstressed, and fatigued upper traps eventually can cause you to hang your head slightly forward. After all, if the muscle can't function wholly, then it can't hold your body correctly, either. The key is not to forget your neck muscles. The major ones are the: *upper trapezius*, the *levator scapulae*, and the *sternocleidomastoid*. The upper trap runs from the base of the skull past the scapula; the levator scapulae starts just below the back of the skull as well and ends at the scapula. The muscle in front is the sternocleidomastoid; it attaches to two bones, the breast bone and collarbone. This thick muscle lifts the chin to your chest and moves your head from side to side.

A stiff neck boils down to this: stress and weak neck muscles. Toned and flexible neck muscles help keep the head in its right place, which is directly over your shoulders. So, if you spend your day leaning over a desk, then stretch the neck muscles every hour. And find ways to tame your tension. Take a stress-management class or practice breathing techniques. Finally, you've got to strengthen these muscles.

So you've got to figure out a way to combat the stress and strengthen and stretch the muscles in your neck as well as your upper back. Easy enough.

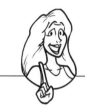

Pilates Lingo

There are three major neck muscles: the **upper trapezius,** which runs from the base of the skull past the scapula; the **levator scapulae,** which starts just below the back of the skull and ends at the scapula; and the **sternocleidomastoid,** which attaches to two bones in the front of your body, the breast bone and the clavicle.

Muscle, Not Momentum!

Okay, upper back muscles are overworked, so how are the joints in your shoulders affected? After all, toned muscles protect the joints. The shoulder joint has an unusual anatomical structure; it is geared to give you a wide range of motion and greater flexibility. You can weight-train to reach for a crying baby or to lift heavy boxes. We use our arms so frequently often taking them for granted, until we feel a little twinge in the shoulder.

What's going on? Pent-up tension, lack of flexibility and strength, along with rapid sloppy movements make this joint susceptible to injury.

If a muscle is constricted, then it can't enjoy a full range of movement and flexibility. If it's weak, then another muscle will compensate. If it's sloppy and fast in movements, then eventually the muscle will give out. You'll always come back to the guiding principles: Smooth, controlled movement is more effective and less stressful on the joints than a wild, uncontrolled, large movement. In other words, use the muscle, not momentum.

The shoulder girdle is a complex combination of ligaments, tendons, and muscles that protect a group of joints; it's a good size starting with the clavicle, the shoulder blades, the upper arm bones, and the ribcage. The primary function is to connect the arms to the trunk. Your shoulder girdle is held in place by muscles. And it gets its strength from muscles, which is why you must work the muscles evenly and correctly. For example, you don't want to lift weight if your shoulders are glued to your ears.

As you know, there are deep stabilizing muscles as well as movement muscles. The deep rotator cuff muscles give stability to the shoulders: the *subscapularis, supraspinatus, infraspinatus,* and *teres minor.* These muscles encircle the shoulder joint. You can feel these muscles rotating your shoulders in and out. With strong rotators, the large muscle movers can do their job with ease and without injury.

Major movement muscles of the arm include the biceps and triceps. It's easy to train your biceps because they're sitting on the top portion of your arm. Now feel the muscle in the back of your arm. That's the triceps group. We often neglect them, and for that reason these are the first to turn flabby. The flab waves long after you're done saying good-bye!

The other muscles include the shoulder muscles or *deltoids* (delts, for short). Then there's the chest muscles, the *pectoralis major* and *minor*. On your back are a few big muscle groups: the *trapezius*, which is divided into the upper and lower traps; the *rhomboids* are located between your shoulder blades; the *latissimus dorsi* is the largest back muscle; and, finally, the *serratus anterior,* which is the muscle underneath your armpits. Strengthen these muscles evenly and you're on your way to better posture.

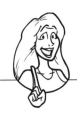

Pilates Lingo

The shoulder girdle is stabilized by a group of muscles called the rotator cuff, or shoulder rotators, for short. These muscles—the **subscapularis, supraspinatus, infraspinatus,** and **teres minor**—encircle the shoulder joint so that the large movement muscles can move with ease.

Leaning into the Wind

Just because you're working the arms doesn't mean that your legs won't work also. You're aiming for tone in your legs and lots of work in abs to support your torso. Let go of your tension, and unlock your joints, lengthen the spine, relax the shoulders, and align your neck so that it's free and over your shoulders.

To do your standing arm work, find a mirror and then follow these steps:

1. Get in your Pilates "V." Remember, heels are glued together and your toes are about three fingers apart. Legs are straight, but your knees are never locked. Balance your weight evenly between your feet.

2. Create a long spine by lengthening out of the top of your head, as if someone has lifted you up by your head. Then scoop your navel to the spine to create a stable center.

3. Imagine the wind blowing in your face; it's hurricane force. To stand tall and stable, you have to lean into the wind and remain rigid from the base of your pelvis to the top of your head, scooping your navel to your spine the whole time in conjunction with pinching your butt cheeks. Think about putting a thousand-dollar bill between your cheeks, and squeeze it. The more your powerhouse works, the more stable you will be.

4. Hang your shoulders. Remind yourself over and over again, pits to your hips. But don't pull your shoulders back; it's a natural hang from the shoulder sockets. Don't worry if they naturally hang slightly forward; however, don't force them back.

5. As you lean into the wind, the tendency is to hang your neck forward, as if you have a dreadful double-chin. Don't. Keep your chin parallel to the floor, and tighten your torso.

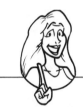

Pilates Lingo

Just because you're working the arms doesn't mean the legs can't work as well. **Leaning into the wind** is an action that gives you a total body workout; you can strengthen from head to toe!

After you've mastered *leaning into the wind,* rise up to your toes, keeping your heels together. That's right, you can do the Arm Series on your toes if you need a little extra oomph, lowering the heels on the last exercise. Besides getting a great workout, you're building your balance.

Jiggy-Free: The Standing Arms Series

Do the Standing Arms Series at the beginning or end of your Mat workout. Anyone can do this series, and all you need is a pair of 1- to 3-pound dumbbells. For example, this is great for the older set who needs to strengthen the upper back, or the pregnant woman who needs pain relief for her aching back.

As with every exercise, you're stabilizing the body against movement. Focus on the shoulder joints; it's muscles and your form. Work to tone the muscles around the joint without stressing the joint itself, meaning no momentum. Don't forget about the principle of self-resistance: Add resistance in both directions to get the most out of your workout. As always, review your mental checklists along with these directions:

➤ Pits to your hips; don't force your shoulders back.

➤ Make sure that your shoulders are even; one shoulder shouldn't be higher than the other.

➤ No tensing anywhere.

➤ Engage in slow and controlled movements instead of big movements driven by momentum.

➤ Don't hang your head forward.

➤ Keep your wrists straight at all times.

➤ And don't grip your dumbbells, because this causes needless tension.

Even if you're sculpting your back to show it off in the hottest halter-top, know this: By strengthening your upper back, you'll improve your posture and protect yourself from injury. So follow the directions to do the Standing Arms Series:

➤ Bicep Curls Front

➤ Boxing

➤ Flat-Back Fly

➤ Zip-Ups

➤ Arm Circles

➤ Chest Expansion

➤ Side Arm Stretch

Basic Biceps

Okay, Biceps Curl, no brainer! However, this exercise is often done incorrectly. Elbows fly, the torso rocks, the shoulders levitate, and the arms swing back and forth. These are all no-nos.

Think stabilization! Work the biceps without jerking your trunk up and down—stay stable. Glue your elbows to your rib cage, press your shoulders to your hips, and slow down to isolate the biceps muscle.

You'll do one set of biceps curl and work your powerhouse. You'll curl in what's called the *Pilates box*, meaning that your limbs should not work wider than the shoulders and hips.

Do the basic Biceps Curls in these steps:

1. In your Pilates "V," extend your arms out in front of you, at shoulder height and with the palms up.

2. Inhale and slowly curl the arms toward your shoulders. Keep your wrists straight, and don't grip the dumbbells.

3. Exhale and return your arms to the starting position. Remember, self-resistance! Keep the elbows in place and shoulders down. You're going for length, so reach your fingertips as far away from your face as possible, self-resisting in both directions. Do 10 reps.

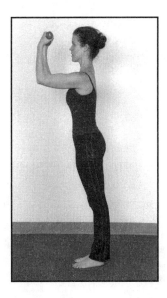

Boxing

For this exercise, you're still incorporating a few muscle groups: the triceps, delts, rotators, and biceps. Let's back up for a second. Think back to the shoulder girdle. Picture the shoulder rotators; they're deep. The deltoid muscles are superficial—you can feel them—and are divided into three muscles to support the shoulder: front or anterior, middle or medial, and back or posterior. You're working the back deltoid and triceps.

Test your Boxing in these steps:

1. Get in a squat position, with knees in line with your heels, and knees directly beneath your hips.

2. Sit on the back of your heels so that you feel the muscles in your legs work. No flab hangs over your waistband, and scoop your navel to the spine.

3. Flatten your back. Look down at the floor so that your head is in line with the spine. Dangle your arms in front of you. With your hands, palms in, draw your arms to the rib cage; elbows are glued to your ribs.

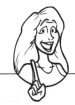

Pilates Lingo

The **Pilates box** refers to working within the boundaries of your torso, no wider than your shoulders and hips.

4. Inhale and lift your right arm in front of your body as the left arm extends back. Move within your Pilates box.

5. Exhale and return the starting position; draw your arms to the rib cage, and the elbows shave your ribs.

6. Inhale and repeat directions as you extend the left arm out while the right arm lengthens back. Do 10 reps.

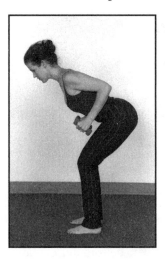
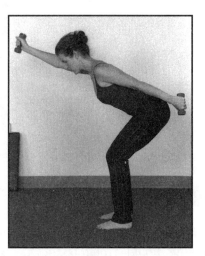

Pilates Primer

Always apply the guiding principles: Smooth, controlled movement is more effective and less stressful on the joints than a wild, uncontrolled, large movement. Use muscle, not momentum.

Develop Your Delts

With this exercise, the tendency is to lift higher than your shoulder height. Watch for shoulder unevenness and belly bulge. As you work with a flat back, the tummy may bulge out. Remember, scoop the navel to the spine the whole time. The focus is the rear delts and rhomboid group.

Do the Fly in these steps:

1. Get in a squat position, with your knees in line with your heels and directly beneath your hips.

2. Sit on the back of your heels so that you feel the muscles in your legs work. Don't let your flab hang over your waistband. Scoop your navel to the spine.

3. Flatten your back. Look down at the floor so that your head and neck are in line with the spine. Dangle your hands in front, palms in.

4. Inhale to lift your arms out to the side; keep them even. Crack an imaginary walnut between your shoulder blades to work the rhomboids. Exhale down. Do 10 reps.

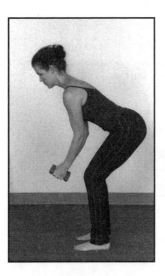 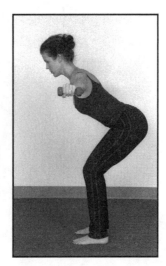

Pump It Up: Zip-Ups

You've probably heard of an "upright row." Here's the same exercise, only it's called a Zip-Up. This exercise targets the middle deltoid, among other muscles such as the rhomboids, the trapezius, and the upper and back area of arms. What makes this exercise a little more difficult is that your shoulders tend to lift with your arms. Focus on stabilizing your shoulders by pressing your shoulders down before lifting.

Do a Zip-Up in these steps:

1. In the Pilates "V," drop your hands so that they rest in front of your thighs, with palms down in a narrow grip.

2. Inhale, and bend your elbows to lift the dumbbells following your center line. Imagine zipping up your jeans, and just keep going.

3. Exhale and lower the hands to your pubic bone, resisting gravity on the way down. Do 10 reps.

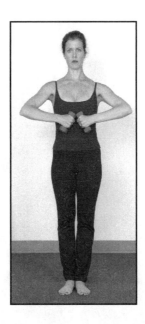

Stretch, Flex, Go: Circles, Chest Expansion, and Side Stretch

Arm Circles strengthen the smaller muscle groups and arm joints that support the larger shoulder muscles, the rotator group. These circles are a wonderful way to release tension and open the back while toning the chest and shoulders, and adding a little definition to your arms.

Make your circles small from the shoulder joints. The sequence is, lift the arms from the thighs to the top of your head in center line, circling 10 times and inhaling every three to five counts. Then reverse the circles and exhale on the way down.

You'll then finish with two stretches: Chest Expansion and Side Stretch. In Chest Expansion, the focus stretch is the neck and chest muscle groups. Of course, the Side Stretch stretches just that: muscles in your side.

Circle the arms in these steps:

1. In the Pilates "V," lengthen your arms out to the side.

2. Open and widen the upper back to feel the stretch. Relax your neck muscles by maintaining distance between the ears and the shoulders.

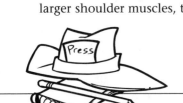

Pilates Scoop

You can always *"relevé"* to make the exercises a little more challenging. In other words, pretend that you're a ballerina, and raise up on your toes to initiate the moves. Then press your heels down as you return to the starting position. Or, stay up on your toes during the entire set to get maximum work and build your balance.

3. Keep lengthening the arms away, reaching out to the sides of the room as you circle the arms up over your head and down to your thigh.

4. Inhale, circling up to the head for 10.

5. Exhale and circle down to the thigh.

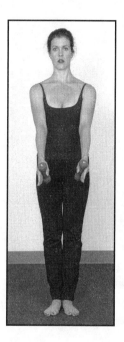 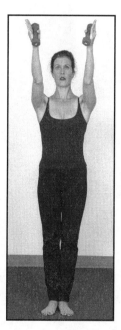

Stretch with Chest Expansion in these steps:

1. In your Pilates "V," extend your arms in front. Slowly inhale and press your arms back, with your palms back, lifting your chest to open it.

2. Still inhale as you turn your head to the right, to the center, and to the left to stretch the neck and shoulder muscles. Imagine holding onto a set of heavy springs as you press your arms back.

3. Exhale and return your arms to the starting position.

4. Repeat the same directions, but start the neck stretch in the opposite direction: left, center, and right. Do three to five reps.

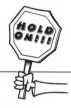

Pilates Precaution

If you feel any tingling in the fingers, lower your arms and rest before trying again. Build up slowly. If the tingling is troublesome, leave out Arm Circles. You may have some constriction in your muscle that's pressing on a nerve.

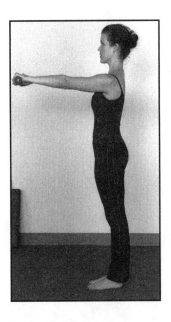
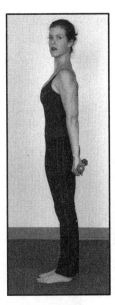

Unbend with Side Stretch in these steps:

1. Inhale the arm up.

2. Exhale over to the side while the left hand reaches down your side.

3. Use the powerhouse to control all the movements. Then reverse the directions—inhale to come up, and exhale to stretch over the other side. Do three to five reps.

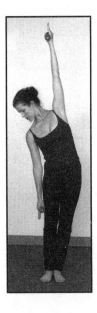

Minor But Mighty

Yes, the muscles are smaller, yet they're important to your frame and sex appeal. These muscles make a big contribution to the stability of the shoulder girdle. Focus on them all to lessen your chances of injury and to keep you looking good!

The Least You Need to Know

➤ Even though the focus is your upper body muscles, you'll work your power-house and legs by leaning into the wind.

➤ When muscles are overworked or tense, there is a buildup of lactic acid.

➤ Accumulation of lactic acid can injure muscle tissues and restrict movement.

➤ The only piece of equipment that you'll need is a pair of 1- to 3-pound dumbbells.

Part 4

Instruments of Torture

Joseph Pilates practiced what he preached and lived a long healthy life, 87 years. When an injured client sought him out, he instinctively knew how to fix the body by using just about anything he got his hands on. If it wasn't available, then Pilates made it. I'll introduce you to the weird medieval-looking devices, and I'll provide examples of the exercises.

Part 4 enlightens anyone who wants to train on the equipment: the Universal Reformer, the Cadillac, the Wunda Chair, the Ladder Barrel, the Spine Corrector, and the Magic Circle. You'll be able to follow traditional exercises designed for each piece of equipment. Joseph Pilates invented this equipment either to fix the worn-out body or to give it a workout.

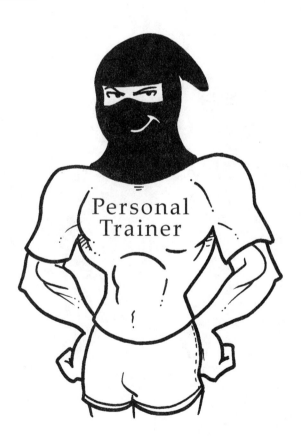

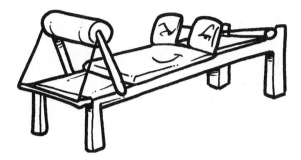

Chapter 13

Body Reformer: The Rack

In This Chapter

➤ All about the Universal Reformer

➤ No weights, no problem

➤ Basic exercises

Picture this: Wiggle into a weird medieval-looking device, wrap your toes—even the little pinky—around a bar, hold onto a pair of leather handles and pull back and forth on a bedlike platform. Sound weird?

Introducing the Universal Reformer. Remember how Mat exercises work against gravity; you must control and engage every muscle yourself. The Reformer, on the other hand, gives you the same results, only with help from the straps, springs, what-knots, and a box. The Universal Reformer enables you to perform a variety of exercises in different positions for both beginners or advanced students.

The Rack: Reform It!

The Reformer is a beautiful piece of equipment. Its sleek, long lines look chic, which is especially impressive because this apparatus was invented more than 90 years ago. The Reformer sits low to the floor in about a 3-by-8-foot space; it doesn't take up too much room. The carriage is a bedlike platform that slides back and forth within the frame so that you can perform a variety of exercises in several different positions: on your back, on your belly, on your hands, on your knees, and while standing and sitting. The dense, firm rubber padding is a nonslip surface that protects you from scrapes and scuffs.

Adjustable bars and leather straps, along with a box, give you a variety of total body exercises to choose from.

No Weights, No Problem!

You no longer have to travel to the weight room to do resistance training. All of Joseph Pilates's equipment was brilliantly crafted with springs; it's the stretching and contraction of the springs that give you resistance.

The springs, unlike Nautilus-type equipment or free weights, mimic the stretching and contracting similar to the work done by your muscles. By using the springs, you can better learn to control your muscles during the movement instead of simply powering through the exercise. The moves are done smoothly. You won't battle against the load of the weights, which could throw off your form. With too much weight, you might work into the joints, for example. Stabilizing your body makes the exercise a total body move. Then you can work the right muscles correctly. In other words, you'll develop the muscles evenly.

The springs are adjustable, depending on how much tension or resistance you need; however, there are certain guidelines. We'll cover these later.

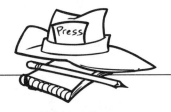

Pilates Scoop

More than likely, you'll start out on a Reformer in a traditional studio because it's the foundation, along with the Mat, for all of Joseph Pilates's exercises.

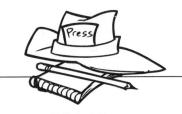

Pilates Scoop

The Universal Reformer is not the most expensive piece of equipment, but can run you a good chunk of change, between $2,300 and $3,500.

Who Needs a Reformer?

Joseph Pilates's vision was to get the body moving safely to feel the substance beneath each exercise. He instinctively knew how the body should move. If it couldn't move the way he wanted it to, he came up with another way to do the same exercise. The Mat was his original work, which he designed during his detainment in a concentration camp. However, the Mat exercises are not easy to do. The Reformer gives you another opportunity to work the whole body in a biomechanically sound way.

No two Reformers are alike: You can adjust the height, weight, and ability depending on whether you're a beginner or an advanced student. All the exercises have a specific purpose and work the body differently. Yet Joe Pilates's ultimate goal was to condition the entire body by using positions of correct alignment and form. Here's a list of benefits of using the Universal Reformer:

- ➤ Works body alignment
- ➤ Improves the blood circulation
- ➤ Builds endurance
- ➤ Develops breathing capacity
- ➤ Teaches spine to the Mat, a core concept
- ➤ Works the vertebrae bone by bone, a core concept
- ➤ Lengthens the lower back
- ➤ Develops the powerhouse
- ➤ Lengthens the torso
- ➤ Stretches the spine
- ➤ Buffs the hard-to-get-to areas: the outer and inner thighs, the bottom, and the lower belly
- ➤ Teaches balance and muscle control

The Underworked Muscles: The Feet

Let's undo the shackles. Take off your shoes and socks to reacquaint yourself with your feet. After all, your feet hold you up all day long. Chances are, though, you don't think much about them.

On the Reformer, you have no choice but to think about them—every workout begins with foot work. Let's go over a few details. The foot has 26 bones, 33 joints, and an extensive system of muscles, tendons, and nerves. Look at your hands; the muscles of the foot are divided and described as the hands are. The big toe corresponds to the thumb, while the little toe connects to the pinky finger.

Not only do your feet support your weight, but they also move you forward or back and from side to side. Just like any other set of muscles, you can develop the muscles in your feet to become more efficient. Your muscles don't always get an opportunity to strengthen when they're stuffed into bulky, stiff shoes. The result: underworked and weak feet. Is this a problem? You bet.

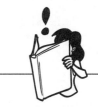

Pilates Primer

Joseph Pilates designed each piece of equipment for a specific reason. The springs, for example, were developed in World War I so that he could work with the patients in their own beds. He actually attached the springs to the patient's hospital bed.

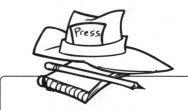

Pilates Scoop

To feel the substance beneath the exercise takes time. Sure, you can memorize an exercise, but the goal is for you to feel it and to move correctly. The equipment used today gives you that: another way to experience the exercise without putting too much stress on the joints and nonworking parts of the body, such as your back.

Our feet are directly linked to good posture because body alignment starts from the feet up. Most of us lift and walk all day long, so the big muscles do get work. The feet, however, don't get worked enough while inside our shoes. Even if we go to the gym for a workout, we still neglect the muscles in our feet. Let's face it, giving our feet a workout is not high on the priority list.

Attention and awareness will go a long way here. If the muscles don't get enough work, then they'll atrophy. At that point, most bodies can begin to deteriorate, to get off balance and center. If we don't stand or walk with good alignment, then eventually aches and pains set in. Healthy posture begins with the bare feet.

Take off your shoes and socks. Stand on a hard surface, such as the kitchen floor. Wiggle your toes. Lift them up, and then slowly touch the pinky toe down to the floor, and the next toe until the big toe. Imagine a triangle on the bottom of your foot. Now, spread your body weight among three points: the center of your heel and between the imaginary line under your big and pinky toes. Plant yourself firmly on those three points on both of your feet. Feel stable and solidly aligned?

The muscles in your feet are now in line with the muscles in your leg. If you're not standing this way, then you're not standing to support the weight of your body evenly; therefore, muscle imbalances may set in. Compare your feet to a car's tires. If one tire is out of line, then it's a matter of time before the others wear unevenly. Your car may begin to shake as you drive it. If unchecked, the damage could lead to enormous problems, costing a lot of money.

Your body is the car. Your frame depends on your feet as a solid foundation for movement. Traveling from point to point is no problem, but the effects may show up much later in life.

Let's say that you roll your ankles out. Your body weight may be displaced on the outside of the foot, a condition called *supination*. The outer leg ends up carrying most of the weight, while the inner thigh muscles get weak because the knees and hips are not lining up correctly.

If you roll the ankles in, the body weight rests mostly on the inner arches; that's *pronation*. Over time, your knees become closer and closer—muscles on the outer

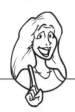

Pilates Lingo

If you roll out the ankles, then you could affect the muscle tone and shape of the leg from the ankles to the hips; it's called **supination**. You may even contribute to the dreaded saddlebag and droopy bottom look as the outside muscles bulk up from overuse.

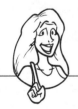

Pilates Lingo

If you turn your ankles in, then the body weight is displaced on the arches of your feet, causing **pronation**. Eventually, your knees get closer and closer together, and your posture is compromised.

thighs weaken, while inner thigh muscles get tight. The outcome doesn't change: poor posture. Neither case is good. You're weakening the muscle tone straight up the body, from the toes to the hips.

Pay attention to how you stand and walk. Awareness is the key to good posture. No matter how bad your posture is, it feels good to you, so you might not be able to tell how you hold yourself up.

So, here's another tip. Look to see if your heels are worn evenly. In other words, examine your shoes. Is one side worn more than the other? Look for wear and tear on the inside arches or outside rims to determine how you're carrying your body weight.

Good body alignment begins with this triangle: Divide your body weight evenly from the ankle and line across the big and pinky toes. As with all muscles, you can develop or redevelop the muscles with specific exercise. It may take some time before you can evenly distribute your weight among the three points.

At first, the muscles will take the easy way out because they don't like change. They prefer to work the same old way—right or wrong—so you have to make a conscious effort to change. Then work with proper placement from the toes up. Think about your feet when you work out on the Reformer. It's up to you to gain balance by reacquainting yourself with your tootsies.

The Total Body Reformer Workout

The following exercises are safe enough for you to try at home (provided that you own one of these machines). However, follow the guidelines for the repetitions, springs, and exercises.

If you have any reconditioning problems, then hire a trained professional before doing this workout. Furthermore, it's not a bad idea to take a private session. A teacher can help you understand the exercises and teach you how to work with correct form.

This workout is a basic workout. After you learn the exercises by heart, you may need a trained instructor to push you to the next level each time.

Get ready to wiggle yourself in the Reformer, for something totally different and healthy for your body as well as challenging for your mind. Here is the sequence of exercises:

➤ Footwork Series

➤ The Hundred

➤ Leg Circles

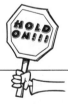

Pilates Precaution

Even though the pictures provide you with a workout regime deigned by Joseph Pilates, you should absolutely hire a personal trainer if you want to recondition your body. You can hire a personal trainer to come to your home, or you can go to a training studio.

➤ Stomach Massage Series

➤ Short Box Series

➤ Knee Stretch Series

➤ Running

Starting Off: The Foot Work

Start by working your feet in the footwork series: the "V," Bird's Feet, Heels, and Tendon Stretch. Besides giving your feet a workout, you're warming up the abs and derriere while gradually increasing your circulation. That's not to mention that the spine gets an oh-so-good stretch.

Two points to focus on are keeping a neutral spine and using the belly to pull the carriage back and forth. Don't bang or lose control of the carriage; it's a constant flowing motion. The back anchors to the bed of the carriage as the shoulders open up. Make sure that the back of your shoulders stays down while you relax and lengthen your neck long. Imagine your spine growing a little taller as the carriage goes in and out.

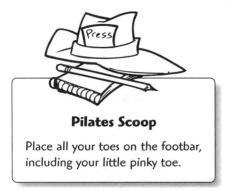

Pilates Scoop

Place all your toes on the footbar, including your little pinky toe.

If your knees lock together or you're bowlegged, place a small pad between your knees to keep them in line during Birds Feet, Heels Up, and Tendon Stretch. Also, don't grind your shoulders into the shoulder pads. If you feel too much pressure, relax—this is supposed to be fun! The movements and breathing are the same for "V," Birds Feet, and Heels: You'll inhale to push the carriage out, working from the tush and abs, and then exhale to pull the carriage using your powerhouse. Focus on full breaths, relaxing the tongue, jaw, and neck. For Tendon Stretch, the movement and breathing are a little different. Put on two to four springs.

Give your feet a workout on the Reformer:

1. Lie on your back with the headpiece up. Shoulders are back and down, and palms are down resting on the carriage.

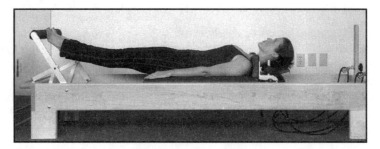

2. Scoop, navel to spine! Toes are on the high bar about 4 to 5 inches apart, while heels are glued together to form a "V." Push the carriage out and in.

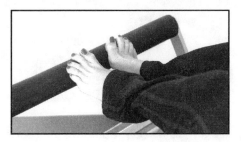

3. For Birds Feet, wrap your toes over the bar like a bird sitting on its perch. Keep the knees together and your feet together. If you can't do this on your own, put a small pad between your legs. Push the carriage out and in.

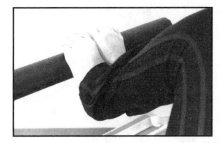

4. For Heels, put your heels on the bar and flex your toes. Keep your inner thighs, knees, and feet together. Push and pull the carriage in. As you come in, press your toes toward your knees for a little extra stretch.

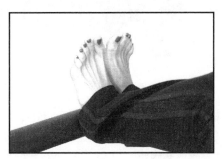

5. Focus on full and smooth breaths, keeping your spine on the Mat the whole time.

6. Finish up with the Tendon Stretch. Place your toes on the footbar, slightly apart, but keep the ankles and knees together.

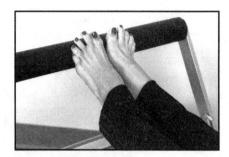

7. Inhale the carriage out, as if you're standing on your tippy-toes. The carriage stays out while you inhale your heels up to your tippy-toes in three counts. Maintain full and smooth breaths the whole time.

8. The carriage stays out while you exhale to press your heels down in three counts. Then inhale your heels up to your tippy-toes in three counts. After 10 heel drops, then bring the carriage in.

9. Repeat each foot position 10 times.

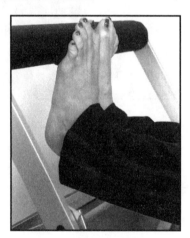

The Hundred

The Hundred on the Reformer is the same on the Mat; it wakes the body up and gets it ready to exercise. After the Footwork series, you'll do the Hundred to coordinate breaths along with movement, increase circulation, and stabilize and warm up your core, only now you're using the springs as resistance. The exercise, therefore, becomes more of a challenge.

Pump your arms while inhaling for five counts and exhaling for five counts. This adds up to one complete breath of 10 pumps, for a grand total of 100 pumps. Or, you can vary your breath, depending on your lung capacity: Inhale four, exhale four; or inhale two, exhale eight; and so forth. Be creative.

During the pumping, nothing moves except your arms. Your shoulders may rock as you pump because you've added resistance from the springs; it's just the arms pumping 6 to 8 inches. Still, you may tire a little quicker—if so, do fewer reps.

Anchor your spine to the carriage to stabilize your trunk. At no time should your back leave the carriage. Remember, you're 50 pounds heavy in your trunk. Attach two to four springs.

Heat up the Hundred on the Reformer with these steps:

1. Place the footbar down, and grab the handles of the straps behind you.

2. Pull your knees into your chest. Lift your chin to your chest, and drop your ribs.

3. As you pull the straps straight down by your sides, stretch your legs out to the ceiling or at an angle. Begin pumping up and down about 6 to 8 inches.

4. Repeat 10 times.

Pilates Scoop

Inhale through the nose, exhale through the mouth relaxing the tongue and jaw as you work the feet—remember, frost the window with your breath.

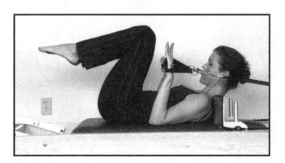

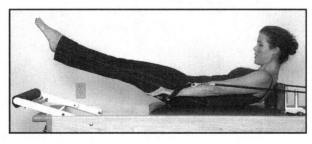

Leg Circles

Here's one for your legs! You're warming up the hips as well, especially if you keep the circles small. Here's the important part: Don't lock your knees. The springs may cause you to press into the back of your knees; instead, make the back of the legs and the bottom work.

The movement is easy—just circle the legs. However, keep the spine in neutral so that the powerhouse circles your legs. Put two springs on for this exercise.

Work the legs with Leg Circles on the Reformer in these steps:

1. After the Hundred, place the handles on your feet. Your arms, palms down, are by your side.

2. Start with the legs at a 45° angle. Inhale the legs toward the body, making sure that your spine is in neutral and that your sacrum is anchored to the carriage.

3. Exhale as your legs circle around to meet back in the middle. Inhale to start the circle again.

4. Do four circles, and then reverse.

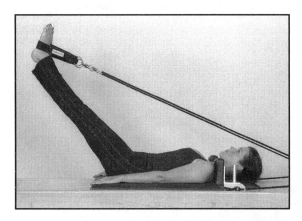 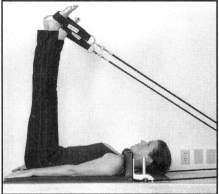

The Stomach Massage Series

Tone your torso! Imagine that your stomach, from the belly button down, creates the letter "C." And, during a good portion of this series, you must secure that "C" for back protection. The good news is, that "C" busts your gut, plus provides a nice stretch for your lower back.

Watch out: Don't lock the knees as you push and pull the carriage in and out. This work comes from your powerhouse. You'll do three Stomach Massage exercises: Round, Arms Back, and Arm Circles. For the Arm Circles, you'll need a pair of 1-pound dumbbells. Attach four springs for this exercise.

Start off the Stomach Massage Series with Round Back in these steps:

1. Sit on the Reformer so that your toes are on the footbar, with your toes in the "V." Hands are placed on the edge of the Mat.

2. Pull up and let your elbows reach long, out to the side. Your chin is on your chest, and your neck is relaxed.

3. Curl your tailbone under, as if someone's fist is in your belly. Think "C" curve.

4. Inhale to push the carriage out. Exhale to bring the carriage in, scooping even deeper. Stay rounded the whole time.

5. Repeat nine times.

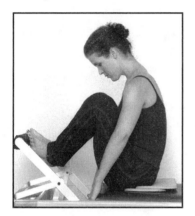 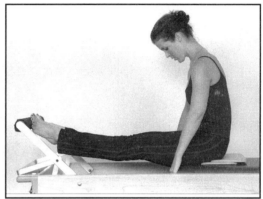

Continue with the Arms in these steps:

1. Sit on the Reformer so that your toes are on the footbar, in the Pilates "V." Hands reach back to hold onto the shoulder pads to open and lift the chest. Be careful, don't hyperextend your elbows.

2. Inhale to push the carriage out, scooping the whole time. Exhale to pull the carriage in. Repeat nine times.

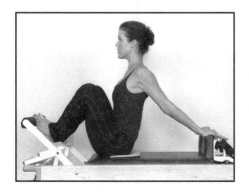 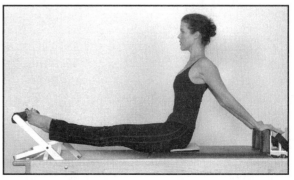

Finish the Stomach Series with Arm Circles in this picture:

1. For circles, place your toes on the high footbar and form a "V" with your toes.

2. With a 1-pound pair of weights in your hands, circle the arms in front of the body, reaching long; then to the side of the body; and finish with the circles over your head.

3. Circle for five counts and reverse the circle. Stay scooped—this is still a tummy workout.

4. And for an extra bonus, dismount from the Reformer with the dumbbells in your hands with grace and control.

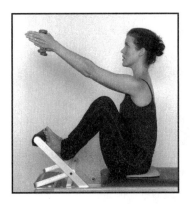

Short Box Series

Another powerhouse series! Even though the focus is on the scoop, you're working the legs and fanny. In this series, you'll pinch, lift, and grow before you roll forward and back. Think back to the Mat exercise Roll-Up. Remember peeling your spine off the Mat? Same concept. You'll round and unround your spine like a wheel, always "lifting" up before rounding over.

Place the box sideways on the Reformer, over the shoulder pads in front of the hooks. You'll do three exercises from the Short Box Series: Fists in the Belly, Flat Back, and Side Bend. Read the instructions for breathing cues and body positioning tips; put four springs on.

Start off with Fists in the Belly in these steps:

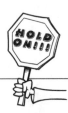

Pilates Precaution

Make sure that your feet are secure under the foot strap. To do this, open your legs slightly, keeping your knees facing the ceiling.

1. Sit on top of the box one hand width away from the back edge to protect your lower back when you roll back. Feet are placed in the strap that is under the footbar, flexed and apart,

keeping the legs straight yet relaxed. Knees face the ceiling. Make sure that you scoop and pinch for stability.

2. Put your fists in your belly. Inhale, pinch, lift, and grow as you curl the chin to your chest to round over.

3. Exhale to curl up to center. Pinch, lift, and grow tall, and then, initiate a 6–12 pelvis curl just like the Roll-Up, scoop as you roll back like a wheel.

4. Finish with pinch, lift, and grow.

5. Repeat five times.

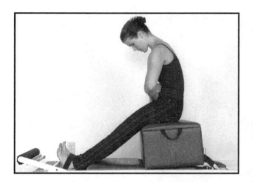 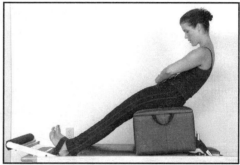

Next is Flat Back in these steps:

1. Reach your arms up to the ceiling so that your trunk is in one straight line. Drop your ribs. Imagine your body wrapped in Saran Wrap from the base of your spine to the tips of your fingertips.

2. Inhale to lean back in one motion, pinching your butt cheeks. Exhale to come up, and then pinch, lift, and grow.

3. Repeat five times.

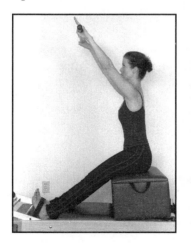 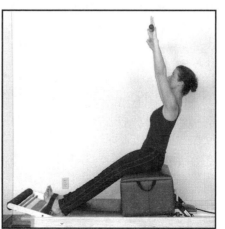

193

Finish with Side Bend in these steps:

1. For Side Bend, inhale to pinch, lift, and grow. Exhale to lift up and over to the side. Arms are placed just in front of the ears the entire time. Inhale to come to center. Exhale to the other side.

2. Repeat five times.

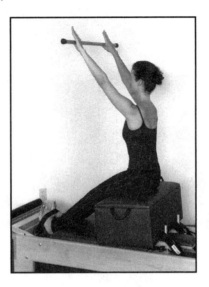

Knee Stretches

This sounds like a knee stretch, but this one is clearly for your powerhouse in addition to your fanny. You may feel a slight stretch to the quad group as well; however, if you feel any pressure to the knees, then don't do it. If you have a weak lower back, be careful.

The exercise itself is fairly simple—just remember to scoop.

You'll see one variation: Round. The emphasis is when you pull the carriage in; you must scoop, scoop, scoop. Don't push the carriage out too far—go about the length of your lower leg. Otherwise, you might lose control in your trunk. As you advance, you can push the carriage out farther. Scoop and stay firm in the trunk while your legs and bottom do all the work. Put on two springs.

1. Put your knees on the carriage so that your heels lie against the shoulder rest, toes down.

2. Wrap your fingers, including your thumbs, around the footbar, opening the arms shoulder width apart. Scoop your belly button to your spine to curl the pelvis. Your tailbone is about two hands' width away from your heels. Float the head down as it looks at your belly.

3. Inhale to push the carriage out about the length of your calf, lifting your upper back. Exhale and pull the carriage in using your legs, bottom, and belly.

4. Repeat six to eight times.

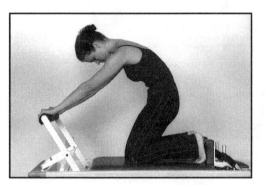 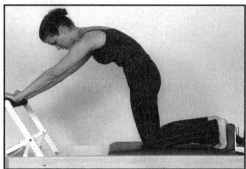

Take a Run: Running

Don't fret—you won't be lacing up your running shoes. Instead, the footbar provides your feet all the cushioning they need. You'll finish with Running. Your knees face the ceiling—no turning your hips out. The powerhouse and glutes prevent this from happening, so coordinate these muscles. Your heels and ankles should be glued together. Don't forget about neutral spine, scooping to control your run. Imagine your feet are like cat paws as they stretch long, displaying their claws. Put on three to four springs. The breathing is a little different here: You'll inhale for two heel drops—lower and lift the right heel, and then immediately lower and lift the left heel. Then exhale for two heel drops.

1. Lie on your back with your toes on the high footbar; knees face the ceiling. Your head, neck, and shoulders are relaxed. Make sure, however, that the back of your shoulders touches the carriage.

2. Find your scoop. Push the carriage out, standing high on your tippy-toes. Imagine the cat's paws.

3. Press one heel down as the opposite heel lifts to its tippy-toes. And the tippy-toe heel now presses down as the other heel comes up. Keep this rhythm, with both legs working just like you're running—one heel presses down as the other lengthens its tippy-toes. Keep the heels together, with your knees and thighs up.

4. Repeat 10 sets for a total of 20.

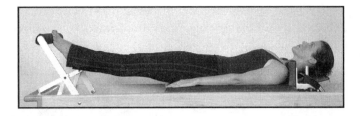

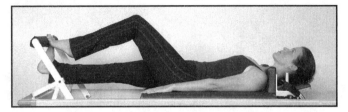

Just Right!

My guess is, you didn't mind wiggling yourself in. The Reformer is fun, and it's something totally different and healthy for your body and mind. The best is still yet to come ....

The Least You Need to Know

➤ Joseph H. Pilates started most of his clients with the Universal Reformer.

➤ Good-looking and healthful postural alignment begins with the bare feet.

➤ The Reformer is resistance-controlled by springs.

➤ A personal trainer can help you get the most out of your workouts.

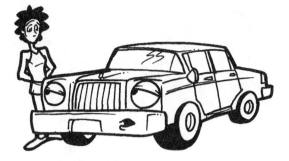

Chapter 14

Bednasium: The Cadillac

In This Chapter

➤ Equipment then and now

➤ Building agility and balance

➤ Reconditioning bodies with movement problems

Imagine a young Joseph Pilates detained in an internment camp during World War I. While captive, he did two things: exercised the healthy and rehabilitated the weak and frail.

While in the camp, he taught his fellow internees his physical fitness program. We know it today as Mat work. Joseph Pilates also treated casualties of war. These patients were either confined to their bed or too sick to get out of bed. But Joseph found a way to exercise their limbs, stretch their spines, and develop core strength while still bed-ridden by attaching springs to their beds.

This inspiration was the prototype of a piece of equipment used today: the Cadillac. You can't miss it if you walk into a studio: It's a medieval-looking bed that has a variety of springs attached to the sides, and a swing that slides back and forth.

The Cadillac provides a great way to teach a body to move, especially a body with movement problems. Whether our bodies need a final stretch or fine-tuning, we should all be grateful that Joseph Pilates thought up a way to heal the casualties of war and that his ways can now be part of our ways—because it works.

Cruising Your Cadillac

The Cadillac is a bedlike platform that is 14 inches long, 14 inches wide, and 24 inches high; it's pretty noticeable when you walk into a studio. The Cadillac is divided

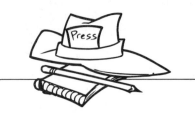

into two sides: open-end and tower-end. You can do a variety of exercises on either side as well as from the top or while lying on the bed. It's a versatile piece of equipment that can challenge everyone from the beginner to the very advanced pupil.

On the open-end side, you'll find a variety of springs attached to the Cadillac. The springs vary in weight—some are heavy and others are light, depending on the exercise and your skill level. For example, light springs are usually good for arm work, whereas a heavy spring is great for leg work. There's also a springlike bar called a roll-down bar.

Travel to the opposite end, or the tower-end, and you'll find a push-through bar along with a couple sets of safety chains and springs. This bar can be either pushed or lifted, depending on the exercise.

In any case, the safety chains and springs can be either attached from the bottom or from the top to offer different resistance. Depending on the exercise, a safety chain is attached so that the bar doesn't hit you in the face. Around the bed itself is a strap. This strap is for you to secure one of your legs, for example, while you do leg work.

The swing hanging from the top poles is called a trapeze; it moves from side to side so that you can do "head to heel like steel" or full-body exercises. Sometimes the Cadillac is called the Trapeze Table. In addition, a pair of fruzzies hangs from the top. Put your feet in them, and you can hang upside down for a feel-good stretch.

Aimless It Ain't!

The Cadillac is auxiliary equipment; it's used to complement an existing workout such as the Mat or the Reformer. Just imagine springing to life after you've transformed your body on the Reformer. The Cadillac is an extraordinary way to finish your workout; one or two exercises later, you'll spring to life!

Although there is no way to show you all the exercises, you'll see a few extraordinary full-body moves along with some stretches. The Cadillac is a versatile piece of equipment. For example, you can use the Cadillac to complete your workout with a surreal euphoria, or you can insert a few extra stretches and exercises to develop your muscles into your regular weekly routines.

Still, you can teach your body to stabilize one part, while learning to move another part of your body. For example, some of the Mat exercises can be modified on the Cadillac until your body gets used to doing them on your own. Or, some exercises on the Cadillac can be used to recondition a body that can't move for itself.

And finally, you can use the Cadillac to challenge your body to move in ways you thought it would never move. The Cadillac brings out your inner child by putting the fun back into your workout, and it's effective. Let's take a look at its many uses:

➤ Improves alignment

➤ Builds overall strength and agility

➤ Increases blood circulation

➤ Builds endurance

➤ Improves breathing capacity

➤ Teaches core concepts in a modified way, if needed

➤ Works the vertebrae bone by bone, a core concept

➤ Lengthens the lower back

➤ Develops the powerhouse

➤ Lengthens the torso

➤ Stretches the body, including the spine

➤ Buffs the hard to get areas: thighs, bottom, and lower belly

➤ Teaches balance and muscle control

➤ Works the body in full-body movements

➤ Teaches you to coordinate your arms as your legs work, and vice versa

➤ Moves the body that has movement problems

No Short Cuts!

Although the Cadillac is fairly safe, it can be a dangerous piece of equipment if you don't follow a few safety rules. For example, you must learn how to control the springs so that you don't injure your

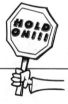

Pilates Precaution

Always start with the lightest springs. When you're a beginner, the springs can be difficult to control, so work on the lightest spring until you gain control, or work with a partner.

knees. Your little pinky toe can get "cut off" with the push-through bar. Not really, of course, but if the push-through bar grazes your pinky toe, it hurts! Finally, you must always hook the safety chains when needed!

Like any other piece of equipment, follow the safety guidelines. Visual safety checks start with each exercise. Follow this checklist:

➤ Make sure that your foot is properly placed on the poles so that you don't graze the pinky toe when working with the push-through bar.

➤ Keep both hands on the bar at all times.

➤ Springs are especially dangerous to the knees and lower back if you work with too heavy of a spring or if you work too fast.

➤ Make sure that the safety chain is hooked first and detached last.

Cadillac Classics: The Exercises

This bed is for you! The exercises that follow are classic Cadillac exercises. You can do them after your Reformer or Mat workout for a little extra work or stretching, or as a way to hone the core concepts.

If you have an injury, the Cadillac can be a great way to get back in shape. However, don't do it alone! You need a trained eye so that you don't further aggravate your injury. Alignment and good form are key to performing these exercises correctly and safely.

Sometimes, when we work with pain, our bodies will often compensate, unbeknownst to us. A trainer watches for incorrect body alignment and movement, plus it feels so good to get stretched out—you definitely don't want to miss out.

Follow the guidelines for the repetitions, instructions, and information on attaching the springs along with safety chains. And get ready to transform your body to "buffness." Here is the sequence of exercises:

➤ Rolling Back

➤ Breathing

➤ Leg Springs Series

➤ The Monkey

➤ Hanging Up

➤ Half-Hang

Returning to Core Concept: Rolling Back

Let's fine-tune the 6–12 curl that initiates the scoop so that you can peel bone by bone. Rolling Back, in other words, is similar to the Mat exercise Roll-Up. Think back to the Mat, and even the Reformer exercises on the Short Box. You rolled and unrolled the body like a wheel. Same concept.

To get in position, work from the open-end by placing your feet on the poles for support. As you roll back, try to scoop even more each time. As you roll up, bone by bone, imagine picking up a string of pearls, one by one, off the Cadillac bed.

Peel off the bed with Rolling Back with these steps:

1. Sit your bottom down so that you face the open-end side, and then pinch, lift and grow tall. Your feet are on the poles.

2. Grab the roll-down bar about shoulder width apart. Inhale to drop your chin to your chest, and begin your curl. Exhale as you continue to roll 6–12 pelvis curl, scooping and rolling down bone by bone until your head touches the Mat.

3. Inhale to lift your chin to your chest to roll up. Exhale, scooping to finish.

4. Repeat five times.

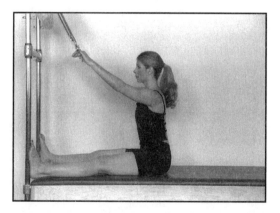 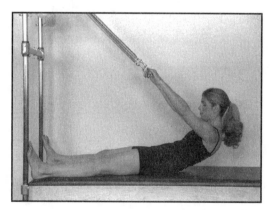

Breathe Right! Breathing

The goal is to increase your lung capacity and limb coordination. Change sides so that now your head is at the open-end. Place your feet in the strap that hangs below the trapeze. You might have to adjust the trapeze so that it swings directly over your feet. Then reach behind for the roll-down bar and secure it tightly.

Let's try a prep: Pull the roll-down bar down. Feel how that engages a variety of upper-body muscles. Repeat three times. On the fourth pull down, leave the bar by your hips. Pinch your butt cheeks to lift your bottom off the bed to meet the bar.

Easy enough. You must engage your hamstrings and glutes completely in union with your abs to stabilize your body.

After you feel comfortable with that combo, try the real deal, which simultaneously coordinates the legs and arms. Breathing was designated to put everything together at the end of a great workout.

Finish your workout with Breathing in these steps:

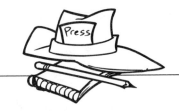

Pilates Scoop

The Cadillac is a great piece of equipment to hone the core concepts: bone by bone, chin on chest, drop your shoulders, scoop, pinch your butt cheeks, spine on Mat, and pinch, lift, and grow tall.

1. Lie on the table. Place your feet in the strap that hangs below the trapeze, which should be directly in line with your feet. The trapeze shouldn't pull toward you or away, but should be directly in line with your feet.

2. Open your legs and flex your feet for support. Hold the roll-down bar, knuckles up. Make sure that your hands are shoulder width, thumbs with your fingers. The spine sinks into the bed, dropping the ribs.

3. Slowly inhale, and simultaneously pinch your butt cheeks to boost your hips while pulling the bar straight down to meet them.

4. Expand your chest. Exhale to lower yourself down to the start position.

5. Repeat three times.

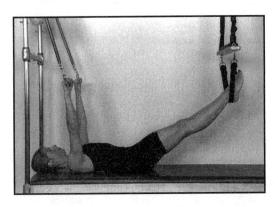

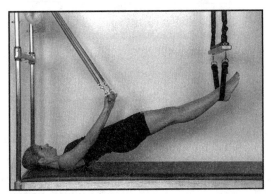

Oh La La: The Leg Spring Series

Need some workout inspiration for your thighs? Here it is. The Leg Series on the Cadillac not only slims the right stuff, but it also works the powerhouse. The secret: the springs! Be careful—don't lose control of the springs, and don't lock your knees as you work with the springs. Turn out your legs slightly in a Pilates "V," and imagine energy out of the heels to make your fanny work even harder.

Work from the open-end of the Cadillac. Your head is just a few inches from the end of the bed. Bring your knees into the chest to put the spring handles around the arches of your feet. Secure your trunk by holding the poles, elbows soft. Then lengthen your legs to the ceiling. Take a few seconds to feel the power of the springs.

Stay on your back the whole time. Focus on your trunk; it will not move. You must scoop to stabilize your trunk, but preserve the little arch in your lower back. Meaning what? Neutral pelvis, with your legs working separately from your hips. Use your belly.

Imagine the legs long—1-mile, 2-miles, 3-miles long while you work. Breathe normally unless the captions specifically give your directions and repetitions. Here's the Leg Series:

➤ Leg Circles

➤ Big Marches

➤ Beats

➤ The Frog

➤ The Bicycle

Kick off the Leg Circles with these steps:

1. Your head is on the open-end side so that you can hold the poles about shoulder width apart. Arms should be straight, but don't lock your elbows. The spring handles or fruzzies are around the arch of your feet.

2. Extend your legs out in front of you about 45°, keeping your sacrum anchored to the bed the whole time. Your pelvis is in neutral.

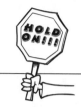

Pilates Precaution

If you have knee problems, you have two options: Don't do the Leg Series with springs by yourself because the springs may strain or aggravate existing problems; or hire a trainer to help you. Some experienced pros use this series to recondition the knees, but that will be up to your trainer.

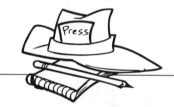

Pilates Scoop

You can also do the entire leg Mat series on the Cadillac: Side Kicks, Beat-Beat Up, Passé, Small Leg Circles, Grande Ronde de Jambe, and the Bicycle. Lie on your side. Secure the stabilizing foot in the strap at the tower-end; put the spring handle on the foot of the working leg, and you're off!

3. Start by bringing the legs toward the body. Circle down to the bed and up to complete the circle.

4. Repeat five circles, and then reverse to finish in the start position.

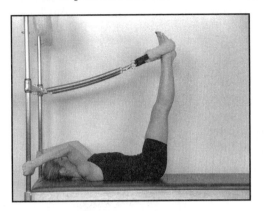 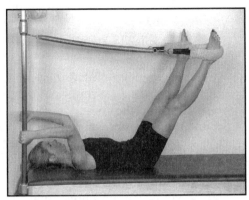

Take a March in these steps:

1. Extend your legs.

2. Split your legs so that one leg almost touches the bed as the other touches the ceiling.

3. Think of shaving a piece of glass as your legs pass each other, feet stay in the Pilates "V." Your toes are in line with your nose, and legs stay in the frame of the body.

4. Repeat Big Marches with both legs six times.

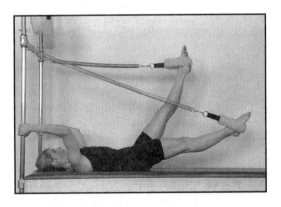 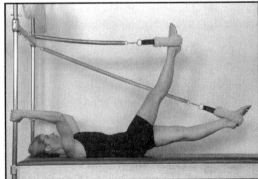

Move into Heel Beats with these steps:

1. With extended legs, quickly split the legs with Small Marches as the legs move toward the platform and then quickly up.

2. Cross the right thigh in front of the left thigh, and then cross the left in front of the right thigh.

3. You must scoop and stabilize your trunk for this one. The legs seal up from the ankles to the hips, beating the heels down to the bed and up.

4. Repeat one set, down and up. Finish by folding your knees into your chest.

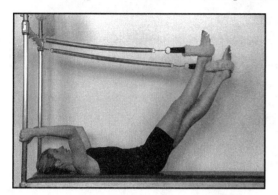 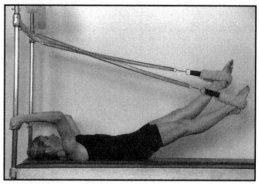

Do the Frog with these steps:

1. Make a diamond with your bent knees.

2. Lower your toes to the Mat, keeping your heels together. The spring is inside your legs. Your pelvis is in neutral.

3. Slide your legs out along the bed.

4. Open your legs to about shoulder width apart.

5. Float your legs to the ceiling, keeping tension on the springs.

6. Close and bend your knees to the start picture. It's important that you keep your back anchored, but maintain a neutral pelvis.

7. Repeat two times and then reverse the steps.

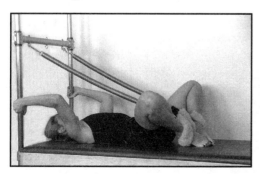 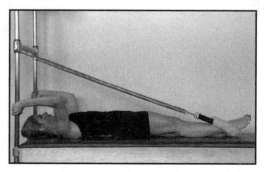

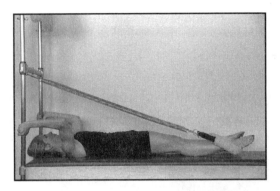
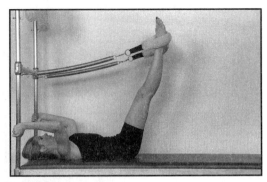

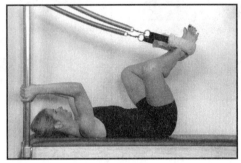

Bike it with the Bicycle in these steps:

1. Extend your legs out in front of you about 45°, anchoring your sacrum to the bed the whole time. Your pelvis is in neutral.

2. Push one leg out and down to the table, as if you're pedaling, while bending the opposite knee. It's important to let the springs come inside the knees, so you may have to open your legs a little wider than shoulder width.

3. Repeat five sets, and then reverse.

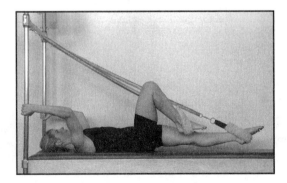

The Monkey

After all that work, you'll stretch with the Monkey; it's a fantastic stretch for tight hamstrings and glutes.

Turn yourself around so that you're facing the tower-end. You have two things to do: hook the safety chain from the top and hook one spring from the bottom.

After that, slide under the tower bar to hang your shoulders off. Grab the push-through bar with both hands, a little wider than your shoulder width. Put both your feet on the bar, inside your hands. Position yourself so that your tailbone is on the bed.

Stretch with the Monkey in these steps:

1. Your feet are on the push-through bar while your hands hold the bar, thumbs with your fingers. Your feet are inside and your nose is to your toes.

2. Remember, chin to chest to protect your neck.

3. Inhale to push the bar up and lengthen the legs, keeping your hips in line with the bar. Make sure that your tailbone is down on the bed. Pull your powerhouse so that your bottom drops even more.

4. Exhale to pull your legs in.

5. Repeat three times. On the third time, lift and drop the heels to get a great calf stretch.

6. Then bring your knees to your chest.

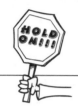

Pilates Precaution

The safety chain goes on first and comes off last, always! When your feet are on the tower bar, they may slip off. The safety chain protects you. And take off your socks because your feet can slip off the bar.

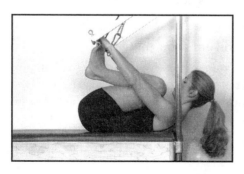
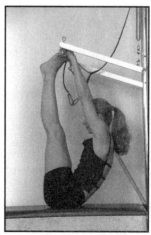

Hanging Up

This exercise is advanced.

To prepare, grab hold of the top poles. With arm strength, lift your feet to your chest and then place your feet in the strap on the trapeze. Then, just hang to form a scoop. And then you'll lift yourself into an arch position, to shine your chest. And then, you can add three pull-ups for the extra challenge!

Hang yourself up with these steps:

1. Hold the top poles. With arm strength, lift your legs to your chest and then place your feet in the strap on the trapeze.

2. Drop your bottom to hang to make a "C" shape. Keep your head between your arms, pulling your shoulders down.

3. Inhale and lift yourself into an arch, shining your chest to the ceiling. Exhale to the "C" position.

4. Repeat once.

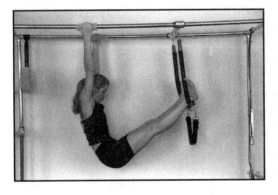 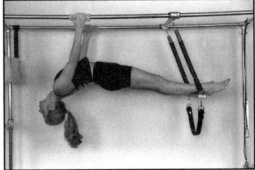

Half-Hang

Here's your reward: the Half-Hang. There's really nothing to this one—getting your feet in and out of the fruzzies may take some practice, though:

1. Slide down the Cadillac so that your head is at the open-end.

2. Grab the poles with both hands, arms straight but elbows not locked.

3. Use your arm strength to lift your bottom high enough so that you can wiggle your feet into the fruzzies. That's how you'll get your feet out of them as well. After that, just hang your bottom so that it rests on the bed. Breathe normally.

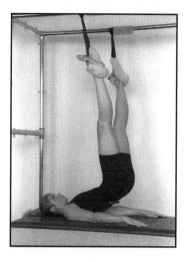

This Bed Is for You

Not sweat dreams, but a sweat workout. Rediscover that inner child, and put the fun back in your fitness with the Cadillac. But hold on, there is more to come.

The Least You Need to Know

➤ The safety chain goes on first and comes off last, always! When your feet are on the tower bar, they may slip off. The safety chain protects you.

➤ The Cadillac provides a great way to teach a body to move, especially a body with movement problems.

➤ Whether your body needs a final stretch or fine-tuning, the Cadillac can give you both.

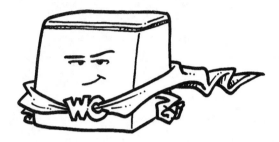

Chapter 15

Body in Motion: The Wunda Chair

In This Chapter

➤ Balance in motion

➤ Supercharge your workout with the Wunda Chair

➤ Balance in and out

➤ Engage your powerhouse the whole time

In 1965, Joseph Pilates celebrated the grand opening of his new gym, which was built on the beauty floor of the exclusive clothing boutique, Henri Bendel, on Manhattan's 5th Avenue. With not a flab or a flap on his thighs, he pranced around in a black tight-fitting bathing suit. He was 85 years old.

His mission: to show the world that his physical fitness works. He performed all kinds of feats on a piece of equipment that looked more like a "potty chair for Pappa Bear" than an exercise apparatus. In his interview with the *New York Herald Tribune*, Joseph Pilates said, "Every home and hotel should have one."

The "one" is the Wunda Chair! This piece of apparatus turns up the gain without any pain threshold because you're balancing the body in motion. The reward: balance inside and balance out!

It Does "Wunders" for Your Body

Some of the Reformer work can be adapted to the chair. However, the exercises become radically hard-core because you're supporting your own weight as you move. The Wunda Chair itself is backless. That means you must engage your powerhouse at all times, making all the exercises total-body ones. The results are priceless: deep muscle control, improved balance and coordination, and increased mental stamina. Here are some great reasons to do the Wunda Chair:

➤ Strengthens the entire body: arms, glutes, hamstrings, calves, legs, and more

➤ Develops balance and control

➤ Builds overall strength and agility

➤ Improves breathing capacity

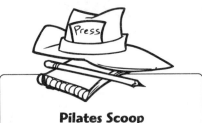

Pilates Scoop

The Wunda Chair costs around $550.

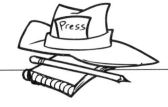

Pilates Scoop

All the Reformer foot work can be adapted to the Wunda Chair: The "V," Birds Feet, and Heels can be done just by sitting on the chair and following the same instructions as you did on the Reformer. The Tendon Stretch can also be adapted; however, it's a little different. The chair is another way to warm up the body and develop the muscles in the feet and on up.

➤ Strengthens the lower back

➤ Develops the powerhouse

➤ Stretches the body, including the spine

➤ Teaches balance in motion

➤ Develops muscle control

➤ Works the body in full-body movements

➤ Coordinates your arms while the legs work, and vice versa

➤ Reconditions certain injuries, such as a knee injury

➤ Challenges the body that needs a challenge

Still, there's another chair worth mentioning, although not featured in this book—the Electric or High Chair. This chair is a little easier to operate because there are handles anchored to the sides of the chair plus a support plank attached to the back of the chair. When working out, you can hold the handles for balance and brace your back against the plank for support. Therefore, the High Chair can be a better place to start for beginners.

Balance in Motion: Wunda Chair Basics

There's no pain, yet plenty of gain! The exercises that follow are classic Wunda Chair exercises. Here's how it works: You can do these exercises at the end of your workout. As you get better and learn more exercises, then you get a complete chair workout. After all, there are 41 exercises.

What makes the chair more challenging than any other apparatus? You're working against gravity while using your powerhouse to balance the body to move your limbs. In other words, these are total body moves that work every muscle at once. A chair workout is like a suspended Mat workout. Although you've earned it, don't be surprised if your body can't do a few of the exercises. You are coordinating several muscle groups at the same time.

If you have lower-back pain, then stop. You might not have the powerhouse strength yet. Work on the other machines, or hire a trainer to show you other variations of the exercises. Also, be careful not to fall off the chair. You may want to work out near a wall for support or security. And finally, lower and lift the pedal slowly with both feet so that it doesn't rebound and twist your knee or grab your leg. The chair can be a dangerous piece of equipment if you don't take special precautions.

A chair typically comes with two heavy springs. On some chairs, there are three hooks: low, medium, and high. Two springs hooked to the low setting provides the least amount of resistance, while two springs attached to the high hooks provides the most resistance.

You know that the spring is too heavy, though, if your knees jerk back to your face—you can't control the push down and lift up. And finally, always face the chair when dismounting from the pedal.

Follow the guidelines for the repetitions, instructions, and information on attaching the springs. Here is the sequence of exercises:

> ➤ Washer Woman
> ➤ The Pike
> ➤ Stretch with Pumping Arms
> ➤ The Jackknife
> ➤ Swan on the Floor
> ➤ The Spine Stretch

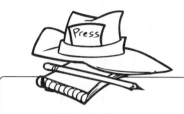

Pilates Scoop

Your body weight, length of limbs, and strength will determine the spring attachment.

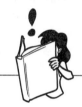

Pilates Primer

Joseph Pilates used the chair to rehabilitate the knee before physical therapy was the science and profession that it is today. Some trainers will use the chair to recondition the knee from minor injuries because it addresses the entire body: feet, ankles, knees, and hips. That's not to mention that many of the exercises address poor body mechanics, which can often lead to injury.

Washer Woman

Washer Woman can be done in two parts: First, you can do stability work so that you can focus on your powerhouse, which actually drives this washer-washer action. Second, you can pump your arms as if you're washing your favorite shirt.

To set up the exercise, stand facing the chair. Bend over to put the palms of your hands on the pedal. Pull your belly button to your spine, which stays lifted. Make sure that your hips are over your heels. This may be enough of a workout!

Here's the powerhouse challenge: Pump your arms three times, keeping the pumps small at first. Attach one spring in the middle or two springs on the bottom.

Wash with the Washer Woman in these steps:

1. Stand in front of the chair so that your toes face the pedal.

2. Bend forward to place the palms of your hands on the pedal. Relax your chin to your chest. Your hips are directly over your heels.

3. Now inhale to press the pedal down, and exhale as the pedal comes up, with your elbows reaching out to the side.

4. Pump three pumps. On the fourth pump, float your arms up, keeping them straight. Repeat the set three times.

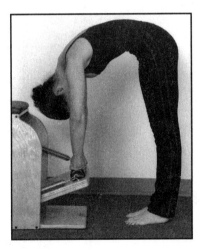

The Pike

The Pike is 100 percent powerhouse, making it a difficult exercise if you don't have the ab strength. To get in position, face the pedal and place the palms of your hands on the edge of the chair, with your fingertips hanging off. Step one foot on the pedal to press it down, and then step the other foot on. Glue your heels together and lift so that you're balancing on your tippy-toes.

This is important: When dismounting, always face the chair and, with both feet, push the pedal to the floor. Then take one foot off while controlling the rebound with the other foot. Slowly let the pedal return to the upright position.

Your hips stay directly over your heels to form a pike position. Don't let your body rock or your hips move from side to side. Hook one spring on top and another on the bottom, or adjust for your weight.

Lift off with the Pike in these steps:

1. Glue your heels together, and lift to balance on your tippy-toes, keeping your hips over your heels.

2. Float your head between your shoulders. Scoop to form a pike position.

3. With powerhouse strength, inhale to pull up in three to five counts. Press your feet in. You may have to shift your body forward on a slight angle to keep the hips over the heels, but strive to lift up with the powerhouse first. Exhale the pedal down in three to five counts.

4. Repeat three to five times.

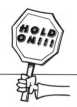

Pilates Precaution

When you lower the pedal, make sure that you lower it with both legs. Step one leg off and then the other. Don't let the pedal rebound because it can jerk your knee.

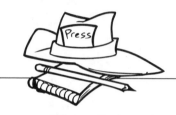

Pilates Scoop

For the super-advanced Pike, try it with one arm. Same instructions apply, but lift one arm to the side. Be careful—you may want to have a spotter.

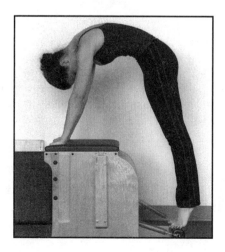

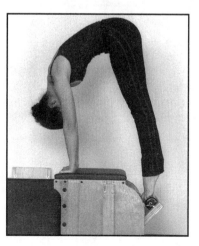

Stretch with Pumping

It's time for a good stretch. This exercise is divided into two exercises: first a stretch, and then you'll pump the arms while in the stretch position. This exercise helps to increase flexibility in the hamstrings and lower back, plus you're working on your scoop. It's great prep for the Mat exercise, the Teaser.

Sit on the floor, and back your bottom up to the chair. Place the feet on top of the chair, and put your hands on the pedal. Lower your nose to your knees to get a great stretch. Inhale for three counts and then exhale scooping even deeper. Place one spring in the middle.

Ease up with a nice Stretch in these steps:

1. Put your hands on the pedal, and lower your nose to your knees to get a great stretch.

2. Press the pedal up and down five times, keeping your nose to your knees. Nothing moves except for your arms, which should be straight. Breathe normally.

3. Repeat three times.

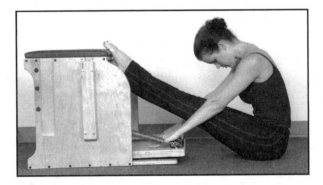

Swan on the Floor

This Swan is similar to the Mat Swan, only you're coordinating your arms as well. This exercise works the back in extension, so it's very important that you focus on pulling your belly button to your spine and pinching your butt cheeks at the same time to protect the delicate muscle along the spine. Hook one spring in the middle.

Coordinate your Swan with these steps:

1. Lie on your belly, facing the chair. Place your hands on the pedal, palms down.

2. Extend your legs out long, pinching your butt cheeks and reaching your tailbone to your heels. Your head floats between your arms.

3. With straight arms, inhale and press the pedal down as you come up into a Swan, and stretch. Pull your belly button up, up, up. Exhale to release the pedal and stretch, as in the start picture.

4. Repeat three times.

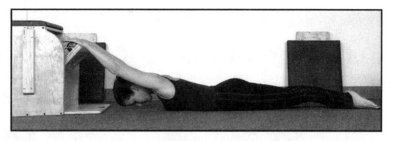

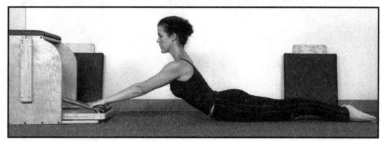

The Jackknife

Here's another super-advanced Mat exercise that can be modified. So, if you can't do the Jackknife on the floor, try it on the chair because it's a little easier. The instructions are exactly the same as with the Mat, but you have the assistance of the chair. Use two springs on the top setting.

Modifying the Jackknife on the chair with these steps:

1. Lie on the Mat, and anchor your spine to the Mat.

2. Hands reach back to hold the sides of the pedals. Legs lengthen out in front of you.

3. Inhale and push from your bottom to lift your hips so that your toes touch the top of the chair.

4. Pinch your butt cheeks to shift your pelvis forward to lift your toes to the ceiling. Your body should almost be in a straight line.

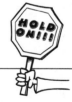

Pilates Precaution

Don't do the Corkscrew or the Jackknife if you have neck problems. Although the majority of your weight should balance on your shoulder blades and be supported by your arms, there is still some pressure in the back of your neck.

5. With your toes over your eyes, exhale and roll down your spine, bone by bone. Control the bone by bone movement with your powerhouse. Legs lengthen to the floor.

6. Repeat three times.

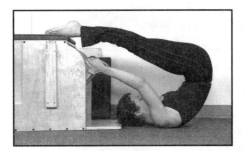 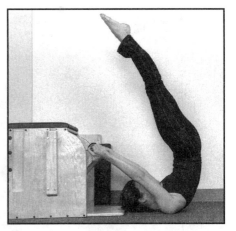

Spine Stretch

Do you see a pattern? A lot of the exercises on the Mat can be done on other pieces of equipment as well. The Spine Stretch is another exercise, and this is how you'll finish up. Place one spring in the middle.

Finish with a nice Spine Stretch in these steps:

1. Sit facing the chair, and separate your legs right outside the width of the chair.

2. Place your arms on the pedal. Inhale and pinch, lift, and grow tall. Inhale for inspiration.

3. Exhale and, chin to chest, roll down your spine while pressing the pedal down with straight arms. Inhale as you roll up bone by bone.

4. Repeat three times.

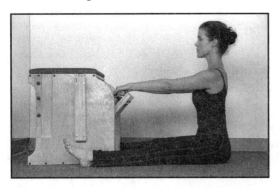 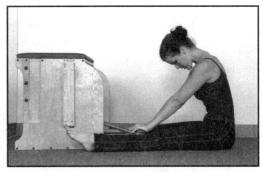

Body Talk

This is your incentive to use your body in limitless movements. If you're not there yet, you will be at least enjoying the process along the way.

The Least You Need to Know

➤ There are two chairs: the Wunda Chair and the Electric Chair.

➤ Challenge the body even more with the Wunda Chair.

➤ You can do more than 41 different exercises, plus variations and modifications, on the Wunda Chair.

➤ You can adapt many of the moves from the Mat and the Reformer to the chair—the core concepts always apply, and the exercises are adaptable from apparatus to apparatus.

➤ Your body weight, the length of your limbs, and your strength determine the spring attachment.

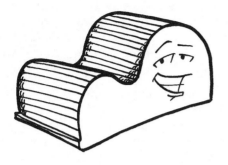

Chapter 16

Spinal Soother:
The Barrels

In This Chapter

➤ Correct your spine

➤ Two barrels: Ladder Barrel and the Spine Corrector

➤ Uncurl your spine

No matter how hard you work at the Mat or how many hours you've accrued on the Reformer, you'll wind down on the Barrel. As soon as you arch over the top, "Ahh" engulfs every bit of your body. The tummy-tucking, thigh-slimming, gut-busting good hard work was worth it because you leave feeling oh-so-good!

Not only will the Barrel soothe your soul, but it can make you well. Joseph Pilates used the Barrels to uncurl the spine and to correct posture. "A man is as old as his spine is flexible," he said.

The Barrel is the last of the big four: the Reformer, the Cadillac, the Chair, and the Barrel. Use the six moves in this chapter to keep your spine healthy and flexible. And then, as the stress melts away, you'll see why it's such a great way to conclude your workout!

Big and Small: The Barrels

Picture this: the hump of a barrel and the rungs of a ladder. The Ladder Barrel is a combination of the two, which stands about 35.5 inches. A slip-proof padded platform covers the barrel, while the ladder and the base are made from wood. There are no springs. No, you can't stash it in your closet, but it's a great way to unwind after a day of stress.

However, there's a much smaller barrel that can soothe your spine and wallet as well. In fact, if you're planning to build a small studio, this piece is the one to invest in first. For example, you can modify many of the advance Mat exercises, which you'll see later. This barrel, sometimes called the *Spine Corrector*, can be just as soothing for your spine as the Ladder Barrel, yet you *can* hide it in your closet. The measurements are 16 inches in width by 31 inches in length by 13.25 inches in height. There's even a smaller version that looks like a baby arc.

The Spine Corrector is safe enough for anyone to use, from pregnant moms to octogenarians to clients with posture problems. This barrel provides extra support for your back by stabilizing your spine, holding it in correct alignment. For example, you'll hold the handles on the side of the barrel and press your lower back against the barrel to keep your spine secure and supported while doing the movements. (Did I mention that it's a great piece to have?)

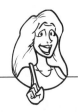

Pilates Lingo

The Small Barrel is sometimes called the **Spine Corrector**. It can be just as soothing for your spine as the Ladder Barrel, yet it's much smaller. If you're planning to build a small studio, this piece is the one to invest in first because you can modify many of the advance Mat exercises, and it's safe enough for anyone to use: pregnant moms, octogenarians, and clients with posture issues.

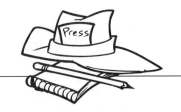

Pilates Scoop

The Ladder Barrel costs around $800 while the Spine Corrector costs around $250.

Baby Your Body

The barrels are used to work the spine to help correct posture, enhance your breathing, develop strength in the arms and legs, and soothe built-up stress with full-body stretches. Here's the connection: A strong, sexy back comes from good posture. The key, we know, is to strengthen the muscles in your back and relieve pent-up tension. The barrels get the job done. Not only can you hold the spine in place to isolate and work the most neglected muscles, but you're also reversing the usual forward bend of the day. In other words, you're uncurling your spine.

The body gets used to working a certain way, wrong or right. Many of us don't unwind at the end of the day. Still, most of us spend our days hunched over a desk, crunched in a car, or glued to a phone. In the end, we go through life crooked and curled. These daily patterns eventually set off a vicious cycle: A round upper back restricts your breathing, which gives you less oxygen and energy, and spinal vertebrae get compressed, leading to lower-back pain.

Our backs are begging to be straightened out. Enter the barrels.

The barrels give your body a break because you get to uncurl the day-to-day grind. For example, the key to antislump shoulders is to work the muscles that hunch over the desk all day. In some cases, working these muscles is hard because they've gotten weak from underuse. That's not to mention that you might not be aware that your shoulders round forward. No matter how imperfect your posture, it feels right to you. The Barrels, then, put you in a biomechanically correct position so that you can unclench the spine to stretch and strengthen.

In other words, the Barrels baby your back and give it a rest from being so busy! Here are a few more reasons to enjoy this workout:

➤ Strengthens and stretches the spine

➤ Stretches the front of the body from chin to the pelvis

➤ Opens the chest for a nice stretch

➤ Develops balance and control

➤ Builds overall strength in thighs and arms

➤ Improves breathing capacity

➤ Strengthens the abs and the lower back

➤ Stretches the powerhouse

➤ Develops deep, stabilizing muscles such as the shoulder rotators and the hip rotators

➤ Develops muscle control

➤ Coordinates your arms while the legs work, and vice versa

➤ Corrects imperfect posture

➤ Gives an overall lengthened look to the body: thighs, calves, arms, and torso

Pilates Primer

The Barrels are used to correct posture, to stretch the spine, and to enhance breathing. You can do full-body stretches that stretch the spine and front of the body from all that ab work. The Barrels are safe enough for anyone to use, including pregnant women, older people, and clients with back problems. There are two different barrels: the Ladder Barrel and the Spine Corrector.

Moving in Place: Basic Barrel Moves

Soothing, smooth moves for you! You'll see six classic exercises on both Barrels. Here's how it works: You can do these exercises at the end of your workout for a soothing stretch, or you can substitute some of the low barrel exercises for the super-advanced Mat exercises. For example, practice the Teaser on the Low Barrel before doing it on the Mat.

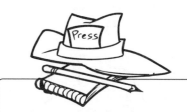

Pilates Scoop

For a little more exercise variety, you can adapt the entire Short Box Series on the Ladder Barrel. Do the exact exercises that you did on the Reformer: Fists in the Belly, Flat Back, and Side to Side.

223

Even though you may be tempted to let it all go, you're still focusing on core concepts. Sure, the exercises are soothing, but you still have to do a fair amount of hard work.

Follow the guidelines for the repetitions, instructions, and tidbit information. The following is the sequence of exercises on the both Barrels:

➤ Horseback

➤ Backward Stretch

➤ The Scissors

➤ The Bicycle

➤ Rolling In and Out

➤ Arm Circles

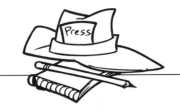

Pilates Scoop

Horseback is another exercise that can be upgraded to extreme by sitting on the box of the Reformer or the Wunda Chair. For example, instead of pretending to hold the reins, you'll hold the straps of the Reformer and use the resistance of the springs to simulate a real ride!

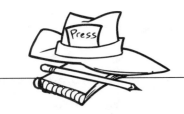

Pilates Scoop

Why the rungs? Joseph Pilates used them to line up the body evenly.

Giddyap: Horseback

Back in the saddle, only you won't be mounting a four-hoofed friend—you'll be using the Ladder Barrel. This is oh, la, la for the inner thighs.

Break down this exercise into two parts: inner thigh work and inner thigh work with arm work. Sure, this ride may be the first without real reins, but that doesn't mean that you can't pretend.

Sit on top and move to the back of the Ladder Barrel. At first, just lift your bottom and hold for a few minutes before sitting down. Then coordinate your arms with the lift. For example, lift your bottom up and circle your arms to the front of your body during the entire ride.

Take a ride with Horseback with these steps:

1. Mount the barrel, sit on the back of the saddle, and hug your legs around the barrel, with your feet flexed.

2. Use your inner thighs to hug the barrel. Pull your elbows to your ribs, palms up, as if holding the reins.

3. Inhale to press your pelvis forward as you hug the barrel to lift your bottom, with light shining through! As you hug and lift, dig your heels

in and point to lift your arms and reach to the ceiling. Scoop the belly. Exhale to come down. For bonus, hold the position and circle your arms in front so that you can see them in your side vision three times.

4. Repeat three times.

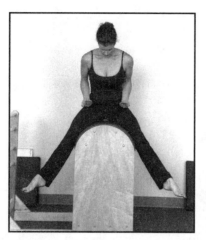
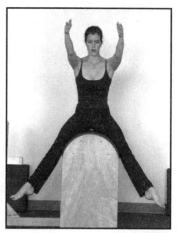

Backward Stretch

Here's the stretch that makes you say "Ahh" after all of the good hard work. The Backward Stretch reverses the usual forward bend of the spine that we do all day and during our workout. The stretch is in full extension of the back—the "Ahh" part. After that, you can flip over and hang like a sack of potatoes as you bend over the barrel.

Go for "Ahh" with Backward Stretch Hanging in these steps:

1. Stand in front of the barrel, placing your bottom against the barrel, anchoring your sacrum. Depending on your height, you may have to use a box to get you in this position.

2. Using your scoop, arch back to grab the first rung on the ladder—relax and let the stress melt away.

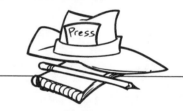

Pilates Scoop

You can do the entire Cadillac leg series on the small barrel: Leg Circles, Big Marches, Small Marches, Beats, Small Circles, and the Bicycle. If you have weak knees or a tendency to lock your knees, the Leg Series on the Low Barrel can be a safer way to work because you're not working against the resistance of the springs.

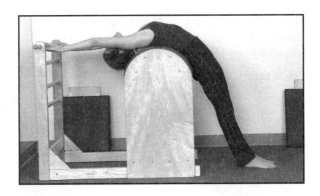

Low Barrel Moves: Exercises

First, let's get into position. Sit in the dip of the Low Barrel with your back against the hump. Grab the handles on the side for support, and slowly arch so that your back is flush against the hump. Lower yourself down. Notice that your chin will automatically draw to your chest. Slither down so that your sacrum rests on the apex of the barrel; it will never leave that spot. After that, anchor the base of your head and shoulders into the floor.

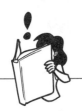

Pilates Primer

Joseph says, "You're as old as your spine is flexible."

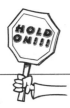

Pilates Precaution

When working on the Low Barrel, you must anchor your sacrum to the barrel the whole time. Use the handles on the side for support.

The Scissors, the Bicycle, and Rolling In and Out

Maintaining quiet hips is still the rule. Core stability is so important in these exercises. Nothing moves but your legs. Here's the good news: With the Spine Corrector, you can build core stability to get you to the point where you can do these exercises on your own.

Just as with the Mat, the sequence starts with the Scissors and the Bicycle, and you'll finish with Rolling In and Out to stretch. Follow the pictures for the step-by-step instructions. The moves are rhythmic, so try not to stop. However, stop if you need to readjust the barrel, never compromising safety for the exercise.

Think about opposition. For example, with the support of the Spine Corrector, you can lengthen your legs to the barrel itself, reaching to the floor each time to really feel your derriere work. However, don't take the extra-advanced step unless you have powerhouse control and coordination.

Do three sets each: the Scissors, the Bicycle, a reverse Bicycle, and Rolling In and Out.

Perfect your Scissors with these steps:

1. Get in position. Maintain core stability as your legs reach long to the ceiling, pinching your butt cheeks.

2. Press your sacrum to the barrel. Stay firm, scoop, and pinch your butt cheeks; it's this connection between your abs and glutes that stabilizes you as well.

3. In a split movement, inhale to lengthen one leg to the side wall while the other leg reaches to the ceiling, staying over your face.

4. Pulse twice and then switch. Stabilize your trunk—no wobbles. Exhale and switch legs in a scissors-like motion, pulsing twice.

5. After three sets of scissors, go right into the Bicycle.

Pilates Scoop

As long as you can maintain your scoop, you can lengthen your legs to the barrel to feel extra tushie work. If the ribs flare up to the ceiling or you feel any strain in your back, then don't work as low.

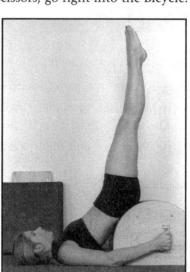

Balance the Bicycle with these steps:

1. Inhale and reach your toes long to the side wall and down to the floor. Then sweep the barrel while lengthening the other leg to the ceiling. Don't drop your knees into your face—lengthen, scoop, pinch, and stay firm. Imagine big cycles as you re-create the motion with your legs.

227

2. When the leg reaches the ceiling, exhale and begin the peddling with the other leg.

3. Finish with both legs reaching long to the ceiling. Then transition into Rolling In and Out.

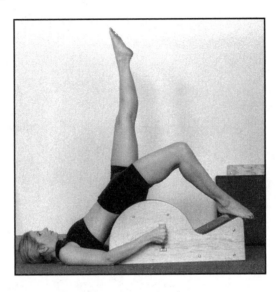

Stretch with Rolling In and Out with these steps:

1. Pull your knees into your chest. You may have to readjust the barrel.

2. Roll your knees just past your right shoulder. Control the roll with your powerhouse. Then let your knees sink into the stretch.

3. Roll your knees back to the center, and then stretch to the left. Move the knees as if one.

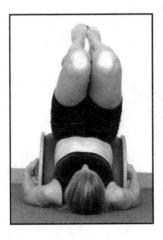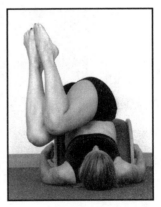

Stretch Over the Barrel with Arm Circles

First, let's indulge in a juicy stretch. Sit in the hollow part of the barrel. Reach back over the hump to feel a yummy stretch as you reach your legs out in front. After that, pick up the dumbbells (no more than 3 pounds) to add a little work.

Circle your arms over the Barrel with these steps:

1. Sit with your bottom in the hollow part as your back and neck rest over the hump of the barrel. Your feet are in the Pilates "V," squeezing your inner thigh and belly the whole time. Dumbbells are in your hands.

2. Inhale your arms over your head, palms facing each other.

3. Circle your arms to the back and then out to the side, palms up. Exhale to finish the circle with your arms in your lap.

4. Repeat three times, and then reverse the circle.

Pilates Scoop

Arm Circles over the Small Barrel are especially great for clients who suffer from osteoporosis or arthritis in the spine.

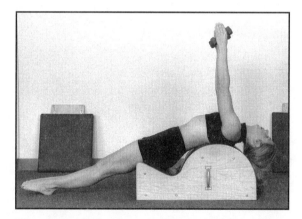

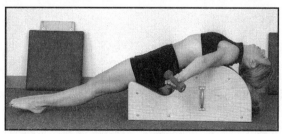

Baby Your Back

After a grinding day at the office, our spines need to unwind, too. Try the Barrels, and your spine will thank you.

The Least You Need to Know

➤ There are two Barrels: The Ladder Barrel and the Spine Corrector.

➤ The Barrels are used to correct posture, to enhance breathing, and to stretch and flex the limbs.

➤ You can use the Barrel exercises at the end of your workout, or you can substitute some of these exercises for the more challenging advanced Mat exercises.

➤ The Low Barrel exercises are excellent for clients with osteoporosis, hump backs, scoliosis, or shoulder and neck injuries, as well as for women who are in the last trimester of pregnancy.

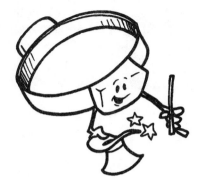

Chapter 17

Simply Fit: The Magic Circle

In This Chapter

➤ Equipment that's cheap

➤ Take it on the road

➤ The Big O

➤ Do it on the wall

Apart from the Universal Reformer, the Cadillac, the Wunda Chair, and the Barrels, you should know about another body-toning apparatus: the Magic Circle, a.k.a. the Big O.

The Magic Circle is the perfect solution for the workout blues. It's small enough to fit into your suitcase if you travel for a living, or you can tone in the privacy of your own home if you can't make it to the gym. In this chapter, you'll get some great exercise ideas so that you stay fit no matter what's going on in your life.

Introducing the Big O

How many times has this happened to you? Despite your best intentions to exercise, you get stuck in a meeting, or the little one gets sick. You have no other choice but to cancel your workout. Let's face it, training with a pro is the best way to go. But many of us struggle with job time crunches, family car pools, and last-minutes emergencies. Still, you may not have the money or might not want to hire a trainer. Yet staying fit is important and is a priority for you.

Well then, you're in luck. The Magic Circle can give you the body results that you so crave in little time and in the privacy of your home. You can do this workout in 20 minutes, which is better than nothing. Wondering why it earned the name Big O? Because it's a circle with pads on each end to support your hands or ankles. The circle itself provides a low level of resistance as you press against it.

Here's what the Big O can do for you:

➤ Strengthens the hardest-to-get-to areas, including the pelvic floor muscles and the inner thighs

➤ Develops balance and muscle control

➤ Enhances good posture

➤ Develops the powerhouse

➤ Tones the glutes, hamstrings, chest, and arms—just about every muscle in the body

➤ Intensifies the Mat exercisers

➤ Travels well

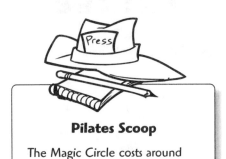

Pilates Scoop

The Magic Circle costs around $60.

Work It with the Big O

The exercises that follow can be done anywhere. Here's how it works: You can do these exercises at the end of your cardio workout to add a little resistance training, or you can substitute the Magic Circle for weights as part of a resistance-training program if you can't make it to the gym. Finally, you can use it to pump up the intensity of the Mat workout. Take the Mat program on the road, or do it in the privacy of your own home. In any case, you can add the Magic Circle to some of the Mat exercises to get a magic Mat workout!

Most of the exercises focus on strengthening the pelvic floor muscles, the glutes, and the hamstrings in conjunction with your powerhouse. Don't forget about the core concepts: scoop, pinch, length, no shoulder hunching, chin to chest, and so forth. By now, you should have them memorized.

The exercises are divided into three sections: Gut Buster, Upper-Body De-jiggle, and Lower-Body Buster. For the first set, do a set of isometric contractions, meaning hold as you count to five and then slowly release with five. Remember, you need muscle control on both the contraction and the release.

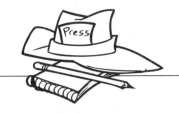

Pilates Scoop

If you travel for a living, then we all know how hard it is to stay true to your workout. The Magic Circle is small and light enough to fit into your luggage. In other words, you've got no more excuses!

Here's a warning: If you release the tension too quickly, then the Magic Circle might pop out from your legs to become a deadly force! Again, go for muscle control.

For the second set, pulse or quickly press in and out 10 times to get a little extra bonus. Then you can finish the third set with either an isometric contraction or pulse. In other words, repeat each exercise three times.

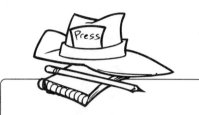

Warm up your body beforehand with some cardio work. Go for a run or take a walk, for example. Follow the guidelines for the repetitions, instructions, and tidbit information. The following is the sequence of exercises:

➤ Pelvic Lifts

➤ Standing Arm Work

➤ Leg Work

➤ Big O and the Wall

> **Pilates Scoop**
>
> The Magic Circle pumps up the intensity of your Mat workout. For example, put the Magic Circle between your legs for these exercises: the Hundred, the Open-Leg Rocker, and the Shoulder Bridge.

Gut Buster

The Hundred with the Big O makes this classic Mat exercise a bit more challenging. Besides warming up your belly, you're waking up the inner thighs and pelvic floor muscles as well.

Remember the breathing for the Hundred: Inhale, pumping the arms for five, and exhale the air as you scoop your navel in and up.

With the Magic Circle between your legs, you may not be able to lower your legs as much. In any event, place the Magic Circle between your ankles or higher if needed, and you know what to do. (If you need to refresh your memory, then go back to Chapter 6, "Sculpt Yourself into Shape.")

After the Hundred, you'll do a series of pelvic lifts, which are pictured. Follow the directions.

Do pelvic lifts with the Magic Circle in these steps:

1. Lie on your back.

2. Place the Magic Circle between your thighs. Put your feet on the floor, with your heels close to your bottom. Your hands are by your side, palms down. Shoulders touch the Mat and are down.

3. Peel your spine off the Mat, leading with your tailbone, bone by bone until you're in a bridge position. Then roll down.

4. Repeat three times. On the fourth lift—for an extra challenge—lift and lower your right heel and then your left heel, and then your toes, left and right! Maintain level hips while scooping the belly the whole time. Feel the glutes, hamstrings, and inner thighs work very hard to support your torso as you squeeze to keep the Big O in place.

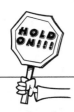

Pilates Precaution

Hold the Magic Circle with the palms of your hands, fingers long. If you grip the circle, you might hunch in the shoulders. Always pull your shoulders back and down to get in proper position.

5. Repeat, lifting and lowering three times, and then roll down the spine, bone by bone.

6. Lie on your back and follow the same direction as the pictures. However, place the Magic Circle around your thighs.

7. Peel your spine off the Mat, leading with the tailbone, bone by bone, three times.

8. On the fourth roll up, lift and lower your right heel and then left heel, and then your toes, left and right! Feel the glutes, hamstrings, and outer thighs work as you push the legs out to hold the Big O in place. Keep your hips steady, and don't forget about the butt tone.

9. Repeat lifts and lowers three times, and finish by rolling down the spine.

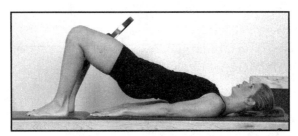

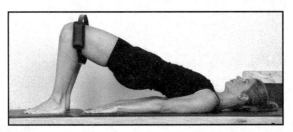

Upper Body De-jiggle with the Magic Circle

This arm series strengthens the muscles in your arms and chest, in conjunction with your powerhouse, your derriere, and the backs of your upper thighs. Think back to the Standing Arm Series in Chapter 12, "Flexing Muscles." Remember the concept of Lean into the Wind? You have to squeeze the backs of the upper thighs, pinch your butt cheeks, scoop your powerhouse, and lean forward so that you don't get blown over by the gusting wind. You'll do the same here.

Tone the arms with the Magic Circle in these steps:

1. Lean into the gusting wind.

2. Hold the Magic Circle in front of you with the palms of your hands, fingertips long.

3. Bring the Big O behind you, palms in. Lean into the wind and squeeze.

4. Repeat three sets: hold, pulse, and hold.

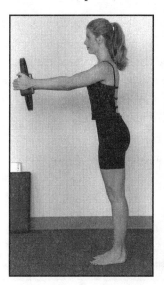 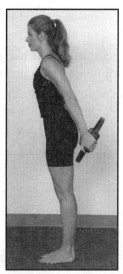

Lower–Body Buster with the Big O

These exercises strengthen and resculpt your backside, plus your powerhouse. This series is similar to the Side-Kick Series; it's rhythmic. Don't stop between the leg exercises, and follow them in order. The transition is a killer inner-thigh exercise.

After that, switch legs. Remember, it's your powerhouse that works to stabilize your hips, so work it!

To finish this series, you'll do an exercise in back extension to uncurl your back from the stresses of the day. Follow the step-by-step instruction because the repetitions will be a little different.

Yes, you'll sculpt the muscles along your spine, plus glutes, inner thighs, and pelvic floor muscles in conjunction with your powerhouse. It's very important that you focus on lifting your navel to your spine and that you pinch your butt cheeks during this work. The tendency is to focus on the Magic Circle rather than to protect your back. So, let's get into a sideline position, just as in the Side-Kick Series. Repeat three sets of each leg exercise.

De-dimple your legs with the Magic Circle in these steps:

1. Lie in a straight line, with your neck, shoulders, hips, and legs in line. Use the arm on the Mat to support your head. Press the palm of your other hand into the Mat, and tell the triceps to work hard to stabilize you, along with your powerhouse.

2. After you're in position, place the Big O between your upper thighs, or your ankles, for advanced work.

3. Lift the legs to the front of the body so that you can see your toes. Squeeze both legs together.

4. Slide the top leg out of the Magic Circle, and place the foot on top of the pad. Put your bottom leg through the circle. Press the top leg down.

5. Slide the top leg off, and put the foot through the circle. Push up with the top leg as the bottom leg stabilizes the magic circle.

6. Repeat three sets: hold, pulse, and hold.

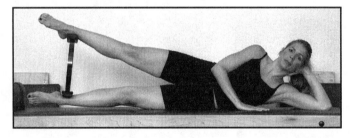

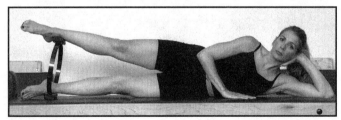

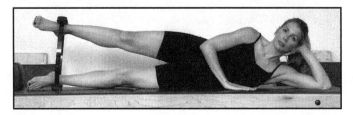

Strengthen the back muscles in these steps:

1. Lie on your belly and bend your knees to place the Magic Circle between your ankles.

2. Rest your head on your forearms until you're ready to lift and lengthen the legs behind you to challenge the back muscles even more.

3. Pull your navel to your spine, and send your tailbone toward your heels as you slide one arm down the back of your thigh toward your knee. Then repeat on the left side.

4. Repeat twice.

5. On the third lift, slide both hands, reaching with the fingertips toward the knees lifting your torso. Draw your shoulder blades down your back. Lift your belly button to your spine while sending your tailbone away from your hips to lift into a slight arch.

6. Hold for three counts. Drop the Magic Circle and rest in Child's Pose.

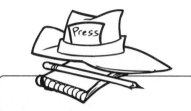

Pilates Scoop

Hey mothers-to-be: The Magic Circle is a great way to keep your pelvic muscles strengthened during the pregnancy, and it's especially great for after pregnancy.

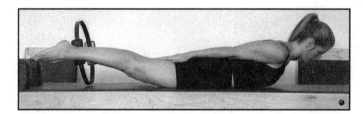

With Your Back Against a Wall

If you find a wall, then you can do these exercises. The wall work is amazingly effective. These exercises help you understand how to position the pelvis at the right angle so that you can work just the powerhouse, not your back. For example, it's a great way to learn how to lengthen the spine without tucking your pelvis. In other words, you can practice your pelvic clocks on the wall to actually feel neutral spine, which is sometimes easier.

Try the pelvic clocks on the wall. Press your head, shoulder blades, back ribs, and sacrum against the wall, keeping this secure position the whole time. Move your pelvis from 6:00 to 9:00. The natural curve in your lower back will get bigger and smaller. Finish in a neutral spine position, but don't let your belly pouch out. Use your powerhouse to lift your belly button in and up, as if the abs are lifting under your rib cage, yet preserve the natural curve in your lower back. So, you get a good amount of powerhouse work. The following are the benefits of working the wall:

➤ Teaches the mind how to feel a neutral pelvic position

➤ Hones rolling down and up the spine, bone by bone

➤ Stretches the muscles along the spine

➤ Drains tension from the body, especially in your shoulders

➤ Works the muscles in the legs, specifically the muscles in the front of the thigh

➤ Tones the muscles in your arms and chest

Working the Wall

What you'll see is a combination of wall work in connection with the Big O—to give you the Big Workout! Follow the pictures in order, and do the exercises one after the other. Here's the sequence of exercises:

➤ Slide Down the Wall

➤ Sit in a Chair

➤ Roll Down the Wall

Slide Down the Wall

This works the upper thigh muscles—plus, if you keep your heels down, you'll get a deep stretch in the calves. However, sliding down is just a warm-up.

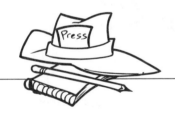

Pilates Scoop

Be careful: If you slide too far down the wall, you may never make it up. Don't go below your knees.

You'll sit on the wall for a more intense exercise and then work with the Magic Circle to increase the intensity. The target muscles are the quads, the hamstrings, the pelvic floor, the inner thighs, the chest, and the triceps.

Slide down the wall with these steps:

1. Stand against a wall, with your shoulder blades, back ribs, and sacrum anchored. Your feet are even with your hips.

2. Bend your knees to slide the spine along the wall, making sure that your feet stay directly over your knees; feet are parallel. Then slide up.

3. Repeat three times.

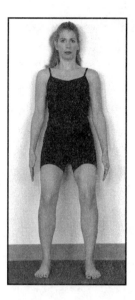

Sit in a Chair with these steps:

1. Place your feet a few inches away from the wall.

2. Bend your knees to slide down the wall, as if sitting in a chair, keeping your feet and shoulders in the Pilates box. Scoop, holding your back flat against the wall.

3. Hold for five counts, and then come up to get the Magic Circle.

4. Put the Magic Circle between your thighs, and squeeze for five counts.

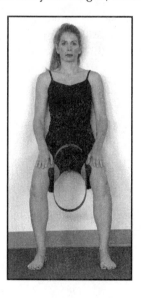

5. Take the Magic Circle out, and slide up.

6. Slide to sit in your imaginary chair; shoulders are back and down. Extend the arms out in front of you, and squeeze the Magic Circle for five counts.

7. Extend your arms over your head, and squeeze the Magic Circle for five counts.

8. Repeat three sets: hold, pulse and hold.

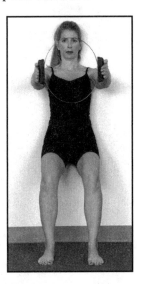

Rolling Down the Wall

Ahh! This is a feel-good stretch after all that hard work, or for after any of your workouts. Peel your spine off the wall and then roll up, bone by bone. This exercise teaches the mind to feel each bone peeling off and on the wall, which is great for beginners. In fact, many trainers will start their clients with this wall exercise just for that reason. If your mind feels it, then the body can better do it.

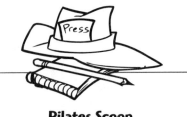

Pilates Scoop

For a quick pick-me-up during your stressful day at work, roll your spine down the wall. It stretches the spine and relieves tension in your shoulders.

Do a Roll Down the Wall any time you need to relax or stretch the spine. For example, you might do this for a midday spine stretch or tension tamer if you sit in an office chair all day. Or, you could do a Roll Down the Wall after a workout. Whatever the case, it's a great way to energize your mind and body so that you walk away feeling alive and healthy.

Roll Down the Wall with these steps:

1. Stand against the wall, with your bottom and shoulder blades pressing against the wall.

2. Drop your chin to your chest to roll your spine down, bone by bone, scooping the whole time.

3. Roll down as far as you can, keeping contact with the wall.

4. Then circle the arms one way and then the other. Just let your shoulders hang, but not your belly. Roll up slowly using your powerhouse.

5. Repeat as many times as you need it. After that, walk away proud of your accomplishments!

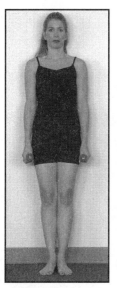 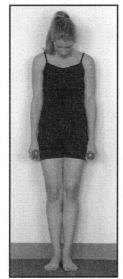 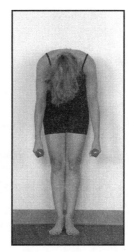 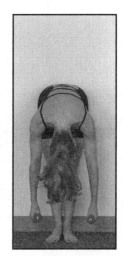

The End

The secret is out—you've been exposed to the range of equipment, plus the exercises that Joseph Pilates developed. Wouldn't you agree that there's a lifetime of moves that will give you more energy, less stress, a better mood, and the finest body yet?

The Least You Need to Know

➤ The Magic Circle was another invention of Joseph Pilates.

➤ The Magic Circle is a great way to keep your abdominals and pelvic muscles toned during and after pregnancy.

➤ Working out on the wall is an effective way to tone your body, plus teach you how to position your pelvis at the right angle so you can work the powerhouse.

➤ Roll your spine down the wall whenever you need to stretch the spine and tame tension.

Part 5

Forever Fit

Part 5 provides you with information about the Pilates world. Are you ready to sign up for the Universal Movement, for example? If so, use this part to get you started. You'll find out what it takes to be the perfect teacher, build your own gym, or determine which style is right for you. So, whether you're a potential client or teacher, hopefully this part provides you with everything you need to get started with the "ideal" fitness developed by Joseph Pilates.

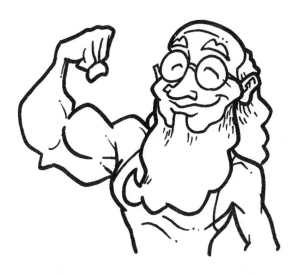

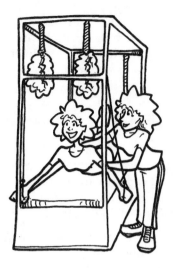

Chapter 18

The Art of Teaching

In This Chapter

➤ Giving life to a 90-year-old exercise program

➤ Becoming a teacher for life

➤ Staying dedicated to the method

➤ Transforming into an emotional leader

"The world needs noble and healthy, attractive men and women! Join the Pilates movement of scientific, individual, correcting and developing the balance of body and mind," reads a brochure published by Joseph Pilates in 1929.

Today, the movement is growing strong. But is it for you? Can you move a body safely suffering from an aching back? Are you ready to challenge a client who wants a hard-core workout? Can you handle with care an older client who suffers from osteoporosis?

Clients need around-the-clock encouragement because some of the exercises are hard. Can you find that balance between a challenge and not a turn-off? Many clients don't know their bodies. You have to teach them. Can you teach the core concepts so that they learn how to stabilize and not work in the joints?

You can learn the core concepts; you can learn the exercises; you can, with practice, figure out the best way to move a body. But will you be fulfilled by teaching? Can you keep the movement alive and growing?

You might be a retired dancer, or you might have taught other forms of fitness. Whatever your reasons for joining the Pilates movement, your teaching influences lives; it's your job to preserve the integrity of the methods developed by Joseph Pilates. As a teacher, it's your job to teach movement and share what you love— Pilates!

Give Life to a 90-Year-Old Method

Call it coaching, training, or teaching—you're giving life to your passion. You must have a genuine concern for your clients, a strong knowledge of the human body, the desire to share what you know, and the patience and empathy to let your clients move at their own pace. And then there's that extra something: a good eye that tells you something about that person, maybe a fact that she didn't even know.

Often, you're an emotional supporter, a friend, and maybe even a counselor. As a trainer, you'll play the single most important role in your client's life. It doesn't matter if you're rehabilitating a client, challenging the super-advanced, or showing the core concepts to the beginner.

A good teacher understands the whole body, from the toes to the fingers to the top of the head. After all, that's the basis of Joseph Pilates's work. Within every exercise, you work the whole body. You're a technician and an emotional leader wrapped into one, driven by the love of teaching.

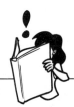

Pilates Primer

The 1929 brochure read: "You can enroll for a 3- to 6-month course. First, you have to take a trial lesson. After the trial lesson, which is an exam initiation, you'll be convinced that (you'll) get results in the promised time. The lessons are given three times a week by appointment, and one hour's work is necessary.

Aiming for Excellence

It's a commitment to be a good teacher. Sure, you've got an edge on the technical end if you've danced all your life. However, good teaching doesn't stop there. There's a lot more to teaching than showing the exercises. For example, you can get other ideas from taking other forms of movement. Yoga, Feldenkrais, Alexander, and even

Tai Chi can give you a deeper perspective on ways to move the body. If you remain open-minded to new ways of movement, then your clients will benefit as well.

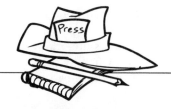

You can suggest cross-training to give your clients a balanced workout. For example, you might recommend endurance work. It's your responsibility to create a well-balanced fitness program for your clients and to know their needs. You have to understand the basic principles of nutrition. If a client asks you about losing weight, then respond with the latest information. Or, if he complains of a back problem, you should have an idea on how to move him safely. If you don't, then you should have the resources available to find the answers. Try to learn everything about training responsibly; it's your job to stay current in all areas of training.

Pilates Scoop

To enhance your teaching skills, stay away from programs that suggest, "It's my way or no way." You may want to attend workouts from other teachers, perhaps even a dance class. Work with a nutritionist or a physical therapist to make sure that you can pass along healthful advice.

Every good teacher has an individual style or approach, but the ultimate goal is to keep the standards of Joseph Pilates's work high. Don't take part in teaching a diluted version of his classic work, such as programs claiming that you can learn the method in a weekend. There's absolutely no way to learn the method in one weekend.

Like it or not, you'll become an emotional support system to your clients. They trust you with their bodies and the end results. Even though you're helping them achieve physical goals, along the way, you're shaping their self-confidence. Successful teachers, then, have a few things in common: patience, a genuine concern for clients, and a nurturing attitude. Show them that you care:

➤ Get to know them.

➤ Teach them something about their bodies that they didn't know.

➤ Design a fitness program.

➤ Be positive and honest with your compliments.

➤ Say it three times.

➤ Don't send the wrong message with your body language.

➤ Know their needs, even if they don't.

Get to Know the Clients

Get to know your students. You can better teach them if you know their health history, their background, why they are coming to you, and their general pressures from work or families. In other words, understand them.

You might end up passing as a therapist. Your clients may end up telling all: their aches and pains, emotional woes or highs, and what's going on in their lives. Just listen; it's important not to betray their trust by sharing their secrets with other clients or by fueling the gossip rumors of the studio. Maintain a high level of professionalism and integrity.

Made to Order: Program Designs

Treat each member as an individual. Based on what you know about the person and your keen sense, you can suggest a particular workout. Designing the perfect workout is what a good teacher does; it's how you will get your client to achieve goals. After all, that's what Joseph Pilates did. The legend is, he experimented with each of his clients and treated each person differently based on their ability and injury. He used his vast, intuitive knowledge to get a client moving.

You can have a consultation, saying something like this: "Based on your background, I see this in you … " or "Based on your health history, this particular workout may be best …." In other words, customize clients' workouts, taking all aspects into account: goals, background, time commitment, money situation, and health.

You probably will have to figure out their needs and maybe their goals, because most clients don't always have a clear picture. What they want or think they want usually has to do with what they've heard through the grapevine. You know, "Pilates is for those who don't really like to sweat," or "Pilates makes you lose weight while you lie down."

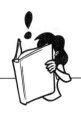

Pilates Primer

The legend is, Joseph Pilates experimented on his clients and treated each one differently. No two trained the same. Through his vast knowledge of the body, he was able to get his clients moving in various ways. He didn't rely on just one way.

Your clients probably want a better body—who doesn't? Yet you might have to tell them that sweating is good and that losing weight is a matter of simple math: Burn more calories than you take in. Sure, Pilates may help, but they may have to do some cardio and watch what they eat to get their desired results.

You might have to work with them a few minutes because most clients underestimate the way they move. Many can't separate the lower back from the belly. As you work with them, ask questions. Use this time to come up with the best approach for meeting their goals and expectations.

With this feedback, along with knowledge of the human body, belief about mind and body training, and past experiences of other exercise methods, you can better design a well-balanced program.

Tip-Top Training: Strategies for the Teacher

Don't train your clients the same way. First, no two clients are alike. Second, that's a lazy way of teaching, which could mean one thing: You're burned out, so get out! Yet, don't design a program that lacks substance. Follow classic method principles and core concepts, for example. You might have to modify the exercise or use a prop such as a pillow, but the method should be preserved.

To start developing your program, you must know a few things about the client. These questions might be helpful:

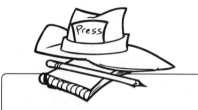

Pilates Scoop

Designing an exercise program is the heart of method. It can be fun, and it allows you to be creative with your teaching and skills. An exercise prescription allows you to better help your clients reach their goals.

➤ Why are you here? Was it a referral? Newspaper? Magazine?

➤ Have you exercised before? When? How much? If so, why did you quit?

➤ Are you exercising now?

➤ Are you suffering from an injury or other aches and pains?

➤ Are you taking any medication?

➤ Have you suffered from a stroke, a heart attack, or some other serious health condition that might affect your workout?

➤ What are your goals?

➤ Are you committed?

After you've reviewed the questionnaire, you can then mentally or physically prepare a program. To customize your potential client's program, you'll use three training principles: Frequency, Intensity, and Time—the acronym FIT.

"F" Is for Frequency

How often should your clients work out—one, two, or three times a week? Frequency depends on two things: money and time. If clients can't afford to come three times a week, then suggest other modalities that will get them closer to their goals. For example, if your clients want to lose weight, then suggest some cardio work that doesn't cost a lot of money, such as walking.

If your clients are dealing with a time crunch, then recommend exercises that they can do at home. Mat classes are a great way to supplement privates sessions. Teach them the basic Mat work, for example, or suggest a nearby class. Mat classes are not too expensive, plus they reinforce principles and core concepts. Let's face it, if your clients get results, then they will continue to come back to you. You should do whatever it takes to make them happy. Of course, you might not want to send a client who is suffering from a back injury to a Mat class; it depends on each client's health and ability.

"I" Is for Intensity

Divide your program into two categories: reconditioning and conditioning. What do your clients need? You should have an idea of how to modify or pump up the workout based on their needs and goals. Healthy clients may start with low intensity, but as the training continues, they will need more of a muscle challenge to get results; otherwise, the body might not change. Muscles plateau, and the muscles get used to working a certain way.

To do this, you might want to increase the load of the springs, add extra reps or sets, or increase the range of the movements. You can add more springs and decrease the reps, for example. Or, you can add more reps and less springs, always making sure that the quality of the movement is good: good form, full range of movement and length in the muscles, and no working in the joints. Here's some other ways to customize the clients' workouts:

To make the workout easier:

➤ Slow the pace.

➤ Limit the exercises per session (6 to 10 per session).

➤ Work on breath control.

➤ Modify the exercises.

➤ Use props such as balls and pillows.

➤ Focus on a full range of motion.

➤ Work with the core concepts.

➤ Introduce the equipment one piece at a time.

➤ Start on the wall.

➤ Educate about the muscles.

➤ Find body awareness.

➤ Keep moves close to the body.

To intensify the workout:

➤ Pick up the pace; make moves rhythmic and add transitions.

➤ Add more exercises: 30 to 40 per session.

➤ Focus on muscle control.

➤ Do the advanced exercises.

➤ Move the limbs farther away from the core.

➤ Focus on precision and muscle control.

➤ Introduce circuits and intervals.

➤ Switch to a lighter spring for core stabilization.

➤ Use all of the equipment.

➤ Use props such as leg weights and the Magic Circle to increase load during the Mat workout.

"T" Is for Time

How long will your clients work out? Most sessions last about an hour, so you must have an idea on how to work them out for an hour, to keep them challenged mentally and physically.

However, you may vary the time, depending on your client's health. Maybe you're rehabilitating a client, so 30 minutes is enough of a workout. Are you willing to do 30 minutes one day and 30 minutes the next?

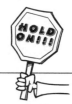

Pilates Precaution

You have to discern the difference between therapeutic exercises and physical conditioning. Depending on the client's need, you may need to design a program with less intensity or more intensity. But you can't train any two clients the same.

Dealing with Clients

Clients like consistency. Yet, you should be flexible enough for change because you might have to adjust certain aspects as you go along. There's not a set way to train. Do whatever gets results.

Keep Clients on Their Toes

Clients need a way to measure their success, whether it's by fitting into a smaller pair of jeans or being able to progress to the next level. Progression is so important because it keeps the student growing, ultimately craving more and more. Growth takes place at a physiological and psychological level. Make sure that you have a step-by-step development progression; otherwise, you risk boring them. Worse, you'll take away the incentive to learn new things.

If a client is coming to you three to four times a week, then you might have to stick to the same program for one week and then move to another program the next week. On Week 3, add a little intensity and so forth. Progression depends on the client, the ability level, and how much time and money is involved. On the other hand, you might have a client who comes once a week. Then you might have to stick to the

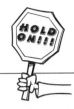

Pilates Precaution

You have to tell the client that some exercises may require a certain level of spotting or hands-on training. You should first ask your clients if they mind being touched. Also check with your state law. In some states, it may be a crime to touch other people.

same program for a month at a time to reinforce learning. Your training methods are not set in stone; you should be on a constant lookout for new and better ways to train. A teacher must learn as well.

No Poking, Pushing, or Prodding

Empathize with your clients as they try to learn new moves. How you place your hands says a lot. You can guide them into a safe position with your hands. When correcting their form, don't push, poke, or prod them into position; it's not about the end result. Teaching is a process. If clients can't get into position, then find another way. Be careful where you touch your clients—in some states, touching may be illegal. In any case, you should always ask if it's okay to touch them, or at least explain that to get better results, you might have to spot or touch them.

Practice KISS

Don't bore your clients with long lectures. Instead, practice the acronym KISS—Keep It Simple, Sweetie! Yes, you must describe the exercise, and you must correct their form, but don't ramble on and on. Collect your thoughts and break down the direction into four to six points. For example, let's dissect the Roll-Up:

➤ Point 1: chin to chest

➤ Point 2: roll up bone by bone

➤ Point 3: 6–12 curl initiates the roll down

➤ Point 4: roll down bone by bone, scooping the whole time

Use the simplest words to give instructions. State directions and corrections clearly and simply. Nothing turns off your clients more than focusing on every little mistake. You might want to focus on one core concept for that session. Pick out two mistakes for that session. And praise, praise, praise the rest of the time. As you get to know your clients, then you'll have a better understanding of what they can do. Keep an upbeat and positive tone when correcting. The exercises are hard to learn, so your clients need constant encouragement during and after each session or Mat class.

Speak their language. Practice prudence as you vocalize a plethora of botherations—get the point? Clients in the learning stages will have no idea what you're trying to say if you don't speak their language. Keep occupational lingo to a minimum.

Praise for Results

Call your clients by their first names to praise: "Hey, Maggie! Great Roll-Up, and the best scoop ever, but work on dropping your shoulders." Tell them what they did well, but don't cover up bad mistakes. Praising their techniques is an effective way of getting them to repeat it. Positive feedback helps motivate them to work on the more difficult skills. Say it loud enough, and say it again. Again! And again! Three times is the rule. Keep the negative comments out. Yes, it's a big part of your job to give corrective feedback—and the sooner, the better, yet not in a harsh, negative tone.

Patience, Please

Watch your body language. Don't roll your eyes if a client can't do an exercise. Hands on your hips suggests that you're over it! Not smiling, or letting out a sigh of boredom only hurts you in the long run. The quickest way to know what someone is thinking is by reading their body language. You can read someone's face and body. It's true—teaching will get monotonous, especially as you train over and over. But you don't have to share your teaching frustrations with your clients. Quite frankly, they don't want to hear it. If you're bored, then you have to find ways to challenge yourself.

Your job is to be patient. Be careful not to send the wrong message. A smile from you will go a long way as your clients seek your approval. Be upbeat, ready to work, and happy to have clients. The message should be, "I love teaching, and thank you so much for your business!"

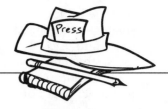

Pilates Scoop

Practice KISS—Keep It Simple, Sweetie! When describing the exercises, try to keep the directions to four to six points. And speak simply so that your clients can understand what you want from them.

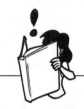

Pilates Primer

In the words of the late Bruce King (one of Joseph Pilates's students), "You have to tell them what you're going to tell them, and then you have to tell them, and then you have to tell them what you told them, and then go back and rephrase it with love and patience."

But I've Never Danced!

"Can I teach Pilates, even if I've never danced?" Sure, you can. Of course, having a dance background helps. Many dancers are gifted with the ability to move and to understand movement within the body. Still, many dancers are exposed to Pilates early in their careers, whether from an injury or part of the educational program.

If you're willing to work hard, then you can be a very good teacher; it's your responsibility to understand the core concepts, principles, exercises, and anatomy, and also to learn to teach. That includes learning how to present the exercises, convey your ideas, structure lessons, and develop program designs for all clients. That doesn't come from learning dance. In other words, a prima ballerina might have all the right moves but might not be able to teach.

Stay True to the System

Ask yourself this: Do I want to spend at least one year learning this discipline? Can I live without income or live on a shoestring budget while learning?

Can you afford to take private lessons? That will help you comprehend the system. Can you financially make it until you build a steady client base? Can you mentally commit to learning forever? That's what it takes.

You need to learn everything you can by taking Mat classes, hiring a personal trainer, reading books, and watching videos. If you're really lucky, maybe there's a good certification program in your area, or you can train under a certified instructor. What you'll do is take a little from that instructor, add a little from that instructor, and then add something new from another instructor. It's a total commitment to learning how the body moves as well as exercises.

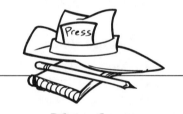

Pilates Scoop

Can you stay mentally committed to learning? Joseph Pilates's original work goes back to the mind controlling the body. That's Contrology.

Although teaching will vary from teacher to teacher and country to country, the core of the method remains the same. You must have a level of commitment to the methods and teaching of it. Every Master Instructor—a teacher with more than 15 years—may teach a variation of the original exercise and have his own idea of how training should be structured, but there's always a high level of commitment to Joseph Pilates's original work.

You can graduate from a certification program knowing many of the exercises and core concepts, but that's just the beginning. Achieving a higher level of understanding takes years, sometimes under the direction of a mentor.

Where the Core Is!

Treat your clients as if they are Olympic gold winners, even if it's the housewife trying to keep her body in shape or the busy business executive striving to regain a sense of balance in his life. Then there's the older set, who tend to need a lot of compassion and support as they do resistance training. Or, the teenager who's battling scoliosis and needs a self-image boost as she reconditions her body. And that's not to mention the athlete who wants to cross-train.

How far do you push them? Being a good teacher means fulfilling your client's goal, not yours. Not everyone wants to advance to hanging off the Cadillac. The reality is that the majority of your clients will want a good workout to feel good about their body and their health. They want to leave feeling like they've just done something wonderful for their body. And you have to provide that because, in the end, they pay your bills.

There's a fine line between pushing your clients too far and not enough: Make the work too challenging, and they won't feel good about themselves and will not come back; make it too easy, and they may not come back. That's a whole other part of your job: to make them feel as if they're doing something great for their health. It's not enough to tell them that exercise is good for the body because, blah, blah, blah. They have heard this before; it's up to you to make them feel it.

Pushing your clients into a set of exercises when they're not ready can do more harm than good. They may injure themselves if they're not physically or mentally prepared to progress. Sticking to the basic principles and exercises may be enough of a challenge, depending on how often you train them and how quickly they learn.

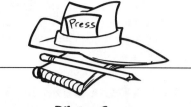

Pilates Scoop

The most rewarding part of your job is to help people get better or feel better about themselves.

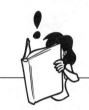

Pilates Primer

Legend has it that Clara Pilates was the greatest teacher. Joseph was the brilliant visionary who created the technique, but Clara could see right through you to help you understand the whole body: its structure, its bones, and how the muscles attach to the bones.

Listen Up!

Your job is to listen and help your clients surpass their own personal goals. Make it fun. You can set goals for them. Every goal or achievement in life tends to be competitive, even if it's competing against yourself. If you already know that your client is the competitive type, then put the emphasis on the process rather than the end result.

A driven executive, for example, thrives on being able to do the move, so do the opposite. Challenge him to the process: the mind/body connection, and the breath and control connection. These principles can come in handy in his everyday stressful life. Don't lose sight of what your clients want, but you might have to create other challenges in the process so that they can't live without you.

Your goal is to work with them to develop further; it's not just about demonstrating exercises. You're improving their whole spirit. As they develop the body more evenly, have fewer aches and pains, and develop a better sense of self-worth, then their worlds get better.

For the Love of Teaching

Does teaching bring you joy? Can you share what you've learned? Will you be able to give a part of yourself to your client? Will you be able to pay attention to other people and their needs? Teaching is a selfless act. Will that make you happy? Because there's really no other reason to teach. Making a difference in someone's life is pretty amazing, no matter how small.

You've got to want to keep the cycle going. What you get from other teachers is then passed down to other teachers, and so forth. Every time you share an idea, it goes round and round, taking on a life of its own. If you can preserve the integrity of the method, then teaching is for you. Teaching takes thinking and dedication—take it from the master teachers, Joseph and Clara Pilates.

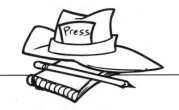

Pilates Scoop

Teaching takes dedication and thinking, which makes it fulfilling in the end.

The Least You Need to Know

➤ You must have a genuine concern for your clients, a strong knowledge of the human body, the desire to share what you know, and the patience and empathy to let your clients move at their own pace.

➤ No two clients are alike, so don't train your clients the same way.

➤ To design a program for your client, follow the acronym FIT.

➤ The most rewarding part of your job is helping people get better or feel better about themselves.

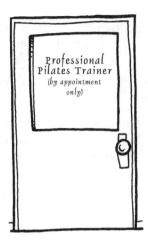

Chapter 19

If You Build It, They Will Come

In This Chapter

➤ Homebody or gym body

➤ Have a business plan

➤ Goals and objectives

➤ What you need for your gym

Suddenly, Pilates is everywhere, in trendy magazines and popular sitcoms. As a blockbuster new fitness, this discipline is being touted as the best workout appealing to the masses.

How does breaking out of the 9-to-5 rut sound? What about embarking on an entrepreneurial venture that merges your personal passion, a healthy lifestyle, and a thriving bottom line? Looking for a few good studio owners.

These businesses are hot. As a studio owner, you should realize that you'll have to invest many steps, plus mega-amounts of time, to get to that point. There will be times when you'll have to work 14 hours a day. Make no mistakes—you and only you will answer to your clients. To see if you have what it takes to be an owner, read on.

Are You a Homebody or Gym Body?

Do you love the energy of a studio, from the clients to the teachers to the movement? Or are you a homebody who prefers working in the privacy of your own home? If you're the latter, then you can transform your living room into a small studio. It's the one thing that you can do quite easily in your home: strengthen and sculpt your muscles. Training people in your home will keep the costs down, and you won't have to fight rush-hour traffic.

Don't worry: You won't need to buy all the apparatuses that'll cost you $10,000, just a few essentials that can give you or the person you're training a great workout.

For example, you can do many of the exercises in this book in the privacy of your own home. You can teach a Mat and offer Magic Circle classes. You can buy a few sets of dumbbells, leg weights, a Mat, and exercise balls—hang a few full-length mirrors, and you're in business.

Or, if you want to train on the machines, you can do that, too. A basic gym will need standard equipment. You can purchase a Reformer, a Spinal Corrector, and a chair for about $4,000—at least, until you build your client base. Then you can purchase the rest of the equipment. Another option is to buy used equipment.

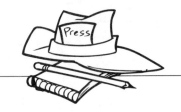

Pilates Scoop

Many studios today are offered in the home. Don't be surprised by the fact that many studios are set up in the home; it cuts down the costs and is convenient.

Gym equipment is a big expense. Again, the equipment you purchase depends on the size of the gym, space in your home, and classes you'll offer. The following list details the approximate costs of each piece of apparatus:

➤ The Universal Reformer: $2,600 to $3,500

➤ The Cadillac: $2,600 to $3,200

➤ The Chairs: $550 to $800

➤ The Ladder Barrel: $800

➤ The Spine Corrector: $250

➤ The Low Barrel (baby arc): $150

➤ The Magic Circle: $60

➤ Ped-O-Pole (not featured in this book): $250

➤ The Wall Unit: $1,300

Just Don't Sculpt Your Bottom, Save It!

Lawyer—who needs one? You do! A lawyer can help you shift through a mile-long list of legalities that must be met before opening your doors. The most common questions include these:

➤ Am I operating as a sole proprietorship or a corporation?

➤ What kind of insurance do I need?

➤ How do I pay the trainers? As employees or contract labor?

Take a couple hours to go over legalities. For example, you might want to ask if it's better to open your gym as a sole proprietor or a corporation. As a corporation, you'll give your gym its own legal identity. One issue is that, if someone gets hurt in your gym, the corporation is liable; the client can't sue you. Yes, you'll sleep a little better at night knowing that your house can't be confiscated. Legally, "incorporated" limits the liability of the individual.

Don't mess with the IRS; it's your accountant who can help decode their rules. How will you pay your trainers, for example? As independent contractors or employees? If your trainers teach at several gyms, then maybe you can pay them as contract labor. Yet, your staff members who work exclusively for you might have to be paid as employees.

As the gym owner, you're required to withhold income tax and pay social security tax if your employees work exclusively for you. But if they are independent contractors, you might not have to pay certain taxes. In the long run, paying your trainers as independent contractors can save you a few bucks. Beware, though! More than likely, an employee working for you eight hours a day won't fall under the independent contractor classification. You'll probably have both if your business is big enough. These are good questions for your attorney and your accountant. They can help you do what's best for the bottom line.

Another critical question is what kind of insurance you should buy. There's a specific commercial insurance policy called a commercial general liability, or CGL, policy. If someone slips and falls in your gym, for example, then you're covered. But you might not be covered if someone breaks his nose if a spring ricochets out of control. That may require a different gym policy. The rules and legalities will be different for every state. Make sure that you raise all kinds of questions: What if someone slips and falls in the bathroom? What if a trainer accidentally hurts a client? What if a client gets hurt while hanging from the Cadillac ? You may need to ask your trainers, especially if they're independent contractors, to have their own personal insurance as well.

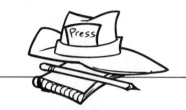

Pilates Scoop

You can always contact the secretary of state located in your capital city to send you instruction forms on how to incorporate your business. The World Wide Web also offers these forms.

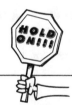

Pilates Precaution

Every state has its own set of legalities. Always hire an attorney in your home state. Ask a lot of questions: What form of ownership should you set up? Is it a partnership? Discuss insurance as well, and determine whether you have employees or contractors. Your attorney will set up the legal structure of the business.

Think of several scenarios to make sure that your butt is covered. You might even have to hire an insurance broker.

Then you should find a meticulous accountant to set up the financial structure of the gym. You'll need to know how much money your business is generating before and after expenses. An accountant will set up a bookkeeping system so that you can see how much cash you have on hand, how much cash you have in the bank, how much money you're spending on expenses, and how much you're producing in total sales.

Business tax law can be complicated and often changes at the state, federal, and local levels. Your accountant can stay on top of these changes. As a gym owner, not only do you have to pay certain taxes on the money generated from the gym, but you'll also have to withhold a certain amount of taxes from your employees, plus pay sales tax from your customers.

Your accountant and your lawyer can work together to make sure that you do everything by the book. Back taxes can wipe out a viable company. And for some reason, the IRS doesn't ever believe, "I didn't know."

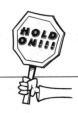

Pilates Precaution

Don't even think about looking to raise money for starting a gym business without consulting an attorney and an accountant.

Moving in? Not so quickly. Expect a delay. That's right, very few spaces are perfect; you'll have to do some remodeling. You may have to give up your dream space if it requires a major overhaul. A good contractor can come in handy at this point. He'll know the legal requirements so that your gym can pass a building inspection.

Each state, city, and town has its own set of legal requirements for small businesses, including everything from how big the bathrooms must be to the shape and size of the sign that hangs outside over your door. Do you really want to spend several thousands of dollars expanding that toilet? These are questions that you'll need to answer before hand-delivering your business plan to your future investors.

No Money Tree?

What's wrong? No money? That's not a reason to give up on your dream. Why not create a *business plan* to attract a few investors? All you have to do is convince this lot—well-to-do friends, devoted family members, or savvy businessmen—why they should lend you enough money to build your dream. Some important points to cover include these:

➤ Why you?

➤ The history of the competition

➤ Defined programs

➤ Who will be your target market?

➤ Who will be working for you?

➤ How much money will it take, approximately?

➤ Who will manage your gym?

➤ How will you promote your gym?

➤ Is there potential growth?

➤ Financial data: How much money will your investors get back?

Your business plan doesn't have to be a lengthy document, but it should be thorough. It's got to answer the big question: Why should an investor give you money? There are entire books, plus software, dedicated to how to write a business plan. You may even want to hire a consultant to go over your plans, your budget, and your financial projections. Write a first draft, answering the questions listed previously. Let it sit a week or so. During that time, jot down any new ideas that pop into your head. Then go back to your business plan to revise it.

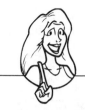

Pilates Lingo

A **business plan** is a blueprint of how you plan to grow your gym. It will tell your future investors what you're going to do, how you're going to do it, and the time frame you'll do it in.

Who Are You?

Besides dreaming of being a gym owner, what will you do to ensure that this gym will make money? Do your homework because you must convince these people that you can pull off your dreams.

Tell them how your gym will make money and what you'll do to make it happen: Will you teach customers? Or, will you hire a staff to teach clients? Will it be your name that is used to attract customers? Or, will you just act as an expert and train future teachers? What will you do to attract people to your gym? Will you manage the gym or hire a staff to manage the gym?

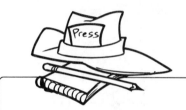

Pilates Scoop

Venturing out on your own may seem far too expensive. The hourly rates for attorneys, accountants, and consultants may seem outrageous. But you're paying for their expertise, which may in the long run prevent you from doing something illegal without knowing it and may save you a great deal of time. That time will be needed for your gym.

If you're teaching, you may not have the time to oversee the daily ins-and-outs of a gym. Who will hire other instructors? Find new business? Clean the gym? Manage the staff? Buy new equipment? And make sure that all your clients are happy? Sound like a lot of work? It is! Sometimes you're a trainer, and at other times you're the manager and maybe even a toilet cleaner.

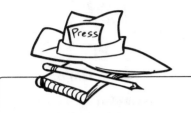

Pilates Scoop

The first thing you'll want to do is register your name, especially if it will be the name of your business. You'll probably have to pay to register it in your state.

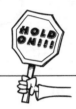

Pilates Precaution

Every morsel of time, energy, and money will be recycled to keep your gym in the black. Know this going in so that you can better persuade your future investors that you're capable of wearing many hats. Don't ever think about starting a gym unless you have realistic expectations as well as the resources and a thorough understanding of the business. In other words, the quicker you can learn everything about your business, the more successful your gym will be.

In most cases, your studio will be rather small. But what happens if it just keeps growing and growing? You'll then have to plan for the worst-case scenario. Employees get sick; some are even dishonest and might not show up to work. Worse yet, you may love to teach, for example, but might not be able to because you're too busy worrying about the daily grind of the gym.

What Are You Offering?

You're still telling about the business. Write down the names of any other gyms in town. Stop by to check out the competition. Call around to see what the other studios are doing. What classes do they offer? Can you offer something different? If your gym will be the first in town, then find out why. Maybe other studios tried but didn't make it. Was there enough of a market? If a lack of interest was the problem, then you'll save yourself a lot of money and time early.

You're thinking, it's just Pilates, right? However, you're providing people with a workout and, in some cases, reconditioning. This discipline can be so many things to many different people. Will you specialize in the traditional methods? Do you want to offer private sessions only? Do you want to provide Mat classes, or a combination of both? Do you want to train potential teachers? Your studio may offer a lot of services:

➤ Private one-on-one lessons

➤ Posture-awareness classes

➤ Mat classes

➤ Reformer classes

➤ Magic Circle classes

➤ Yoga or Feldenkrais classes (perhaps adding other body-therapy modalities)

➤ Certification programs for potential teachers

➤ Spine Corrector classes

Booking Your Clients

Okay, you've got a list of programs. Based on these offered disciplines, you can decide on what equipment you'll need—and, more importantly, who will come to your classes, whether stay-at-home moms or businessmen.

Your goal is to fill these classes and make sure that the gym is hustling and bustling at all times. For example, your most popular hours for classes probably are between the hours of 6:00 A.M. and 8:00 A.M., and 6:00 P.M. and 8:00 P.M. for adults, the off-work hours. At the same time, and during the downtime, you need to still have enough teachers available to train privates. Your system should be set up to book sessions with clients in advance. A monthly class schedule can be offered to all your clients so that they can pick and choose classes and times. Depending on how much room you have, clients may need to sign up for classes as well.

The Big Bucks

Here's the hard part: figuring out the potential profits of your gym, such as doing a month-by-month income and cash flow projection for your business. Do the research. You may want to investigate the market. Ask other gym owners for some guidance. Ask about the profits and the expenses to run a gym. Potential investors will want to know these things before handing over money to you because they want to make money, too.

The A-Team

By now, you've got an idea about the market and the programs, and a general overview of how your gym will run. You're pretty ecstatic because your dream nears reality—at least, on paper.

Look back to the classes. Although you're a super teacher, you won't be able to do this alone. You may want to teach eight hours a day, but, realistically, you may be putting out all kinds of fires. You never know what problem may arise. So, hire the A-team. And that's how your gym will grow as well. You can make more money doing so—more trainers means more classes, more private lessons, and more money.

Even if you want a small operation, you'll need some help to share the workload. A gym can't operate successfully as a one-man show; it's teamwork.

Now Hiring the A-Team

Now you're looking for a few good teachers. Look for people who will represent your gym well. These people should be friendly, courteous, educated, competent, fit, capable, compassionate, and trustworthy; they also should have good values and be go-getter types. Don't limit your search; potential teachers can range from other people teaching fitness to former dancers. You should hire certified instructors only. Teachers invested a lot of time and money to preserve the integrity of the methods and exercises, and they are willing to grow and take pride in teaching.

All good teachers possess one skill: patience. This discipline is not an easy sport to grasp. Most clients feel uncoordinated or don't have the strength. You don't want to hire a set of drill sergeants screaming them into shape. Still, you don't want trainers snickering at the clients who can't roll up off the Mat. Find teachers who will stay a few minutes after class to help clients, if asked. Find someone who will go that extra step just because she loves to teach and is fulfilled by the smiles.

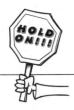

Pilates Precaution

Be careful recruiting trainers. Former dancers may seem like an obvious choice, yet just because someone has the skills doesn't mean that he is the best option. You need a compassionate, kind, and patient person to teach.

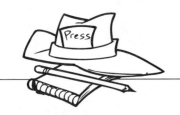

Pilates Scoop

You may be the bookkeeper, while your office managers might also be one of your teachers. When you're operating a small business, the staff members may have to become multitalented.

Your staff represents you. You can have the trendiest gym in town with top-notch equipment, but if you don't have an excellent staff, then your clients won't come back. This discipline is also expensive for the client. A great teacher will keep them coming back for more; a well-informed teacher keeps your studio booming, alive with full classes. And a healthy bottom line will make your investors very happy.

For Rent!

You want a place where dreams are made. How much space will you need for your A-team and their clients? Be realistic—big is not always better. The size of the gym depends on two things: the location and how much money you have. This part is tricky. You'll have to somehow justify why you need so much space and at this location. Come up with an estimate of how much space you'll need for your clients and staff to train safely in the programs that you'll offer.

More services, in general, will mean more money. However, if your heart is set on a space situated in the city's most expensive real estate, then you may have to limit your services, especially if your space is not as large as you dreamed of.

On the other hand, you'll need a lot more space if you're thinking about training future teachers so that they can observe you as you teach in the studio and for offering weekend seminars.

Reality strikes when looking for real estate. You'll find out what you can and can't do. Classes that you originally envisioned may not be realistic at this point. Hire a professional. A real-estate broker will do the legwork for you. Besides saving you a lot of time, in the end, he may be able to get you the best deal.

A key to ensuring the stability of the gym is obtaining the least amount of space at the lowest possible cost. However, you don't want to sacrifice the safety of your students or your trainers.

Field of Dreams

Just because you built it doesn't mean people will come. Pick an area of town that gets a lot of traffic; it should be fairly convenient for people. Some people like to train before work; others may come after work.

You need a lot of people, too. You may have to set up your gym in a shopping strip or near a busy highway. As people are stuck in bumper-to-bumper traffic, they may get the idea to veer off the highway to work out while every other motorist stresses out—what a good advertisement slogan: Stress Out or Work Out?

In addition to finding a highly visible spot, pick a place that's convenient—perhaps that has a lot of foot traffic. Very few people seek out Pilates studios, unless they have heard of the method. You may want to attach your gym to a more established athletic club, for example. Before signing on the dotted line, consider the following:

➤ Find a space that can handle the programs that you want to teach.

➤ Find a location that is convenient for your target clientele.

➤ Pick an area that gets a lot of foot traffic.

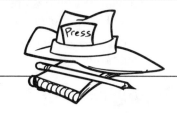

Pilates Scoop

Most studios are small. Approximately 1,000 square feet should be enough room to fit a Reformer, a Cadillac, and a chair.

Pilates Scoop

Think about how much money you can charge your students per month per class. For a Mat class, that can be anywhere from $10 to $20 per class; for privates, you can charge between $50 and $75 per session. Of course, those figures may vary, depending on your state and location.

Start Spreading the News

Spreading the news without spending a dollar—sounds great! Most studios will operate by word of mouth. In most cases, this method will be your most effective way of attracting new clients. That's why you need a great staff, consistently good classes, and a decent facility. Customers do talk.

Why not show off your staff? Give a demonstration of what your gym is all about. You can perform classes in the mall or at private or corporate businesses. You may want to exhibit a Mat class or a workout on the Reformer.

You may want to contact the human resources department of a major corporation to discuss the possibility of free classes. Another strategy: Institute "Invite a Friend" Day. Have your students bring in their friends; you can thank them by giving a free month's membership. Other ideas include flyers, the Yellow Pages, the World Wide Web, exposure at sporting tournaments, and charity membership giveaways. The list can go on and on. Get creative. You can always purchase a book to get a few ideas on ways to advertise for free.

If you've a little pocket change, then you may want to pay to advertise. Design an eye-catching brochure and logo, or set up a home page or an e-mail address. Although expensive, television, radio, magazine, and newspaper ads are great ways to get the word out. The best advertising, though, is to get free publicity for your gym.

Even if you don't have a lot of money, you can always ask a TV producer to swap air time for private sessions. Who knows, maybe you can find a graphic artist who wants to try Pilates. Never underestimate the power of Pilates and the bartering system.

You may need to develop a marketing plan along with your business plan. Marketing your business is vital to its growth. Repeat customers are the lifeblood to any business.

Buying the Equipment

If you're dreaming of a full-featured gym, then you'll have to add more of the basics, depending on how many trainers you want. You'll have to buy enough equipment so that each trainer can train every hour.

To equip your gym, make a list of dream equipment and realistic equipment. You may want three Reformers and two Cadillacs, but your gym size is only 1,000 square feet. When deciding on an equipment budget, make a picture of the space, or get a floor plan from the broker. Then walk through the space. Mentally place a Reformer here and a Cadillac over there, with Mat classes in the middle, the front desk in the front—you get the point. You're mentally designing your gym. Think safety. You don't want trainers and clients rubbing elbows. Teachers need enough space to be around their clients so that they can spot. You definitely don't want your clients jam-packed in a Mat class—the teacher should be able to see everyone.

Nobody wants to work out in a dirty studio. After every client leaves, you should wipe down the equipment with some kind of cleaning solution. If you maintain your equipment on a regular basis, it will last for years. Here are a few housecleaning tips:

➤ **To clean the equipment**: In a spray bottle, dilute $\frac{1}{4}$ cup of Lysol and about 1 quart of water. Wipe off the equipment after every use. Be sure to clean off all the surfaces of equipment: vinyl, wooden handles, the foot bar, and the straps, if leather. Wipe dry with a clean rag. The tracks can be cleaned with a dry cloth.

➤ **For track conditioning**: Once or twice a year, rub a thin film of paraffin onto the track, using the finest steel wool available.

➤ **To clean the springs:** Take all the springs off the machine, lay them flat, and match them according to length (remember, no two springs are exactly alike.) The springs should closely match, though. If the space between the coils is stretched or uneven, the spring needs replacing.

➤ **To clean the casters:** Turn the carriage over, and spin your casters to test for accuracy. The casters should spin evenly and at similar speeds. If not, lubricate them with sewing machine oil. After lubrication, if they do not spin evenly, try switching them to opposite sides. If they are still uneven, you have to replace them.

Finding the Right Stuff?

You probably won't have all the right answers to these questions. The truth is, you might rewrite your business plan several times. It takes time to do the necessary research, and your dream will take on a life of its own. In other words, what you thought you wanted might not be what you want after all.

Several drafts later, after miles of serious leg work and hours of legal babble, you've got yourself a decent business plan. Show it to your attorney; he can make sure that you didn't say something that can get you into trouble. You need a certain amount of money to live on while your business grows. All the start-up expenses include funds for staff, equipment, advertising, attorney's fees, rent, remodeling, and so on. You'll quickly lose all credibility if you've asked for $10,000 when, in fact, you need $15,000 to open your doors.

Your mission: Add up all your expenses and then figure out if you can get enough members to cover that amount, plus some left over for you and your investors. You're building your dream!

The Least You Need to Know

➤ Create a business plan to attract a few investors to give you the money for your gym.

➤ Why you? Think about competition, classes, target, staff, estimated money, advertising, and potential growth.

➤ You'll have to determine your monthly expenses to figure out how many clients you need so that you come out ahead.

➤ Expenses will range from the staff to the equipment.

➤ Hire a good business attorney; he'll work on your behalf.

➤ You'll need an accountant as well.

➤ You can promote your gym for free, by word of mouth and demonstrations.

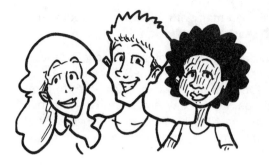

Chapter 20

The Many Faces of Pilates

Pilates is like a pot of Grandma's homemade chicken soup—you never know what you're going to get—but it's good medicine! Is this so bad? Show me two identical aerobics classes, or a resistance trainer who trains like the next one. After all, that's teaching; we learn from a master teacher and then pass on the work with our own distinct styles.

For years, master teachers have passed on Joseph Pilates's work. Many were devoted to Joseph and his work; because of these dedicated master teachers, the original message has spread to me—and now to you.

But we're not there yet. If you were to randomly ask strangers walking down the street about Pilates, then the answers would probably be, "What's Pee-lit-is?"

So, let's define it. It's a method. It's discipline. It's fitness that tightens and tones. It's reconditioning. It's a sophisticated mode of cross-training. It's a resistance program. It's Mat. It's a series of stretches. But, most of all, it's the ideal fitness. So, whether you're a potential client or a hopeful teacher, this chapter is about finding the right style for you.

The Good Old Days!

Back in the good old days, master teachers studied and worked under the supervision of Joseph and Clara Pilates. Many of them were dancers who ended up at Joseph's doorstep because they were injured; it was rumored that he could fix their injuries and get them dancing again. He did and, in return, many stayed with him to learn from him or returned after retiring from professional dancing.

Many have died, but they left their imprint on many of their students. Today the third generation of teachers continues to share Joseph's vision.

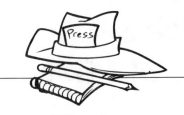

Pilates Scoop

Because of a handful of devoted master teachers, Joseph's method now has broad appeal. This was Joseph's dream for his work. He wanted everyone to accept his ideal fitness. He used to say that his ideas were about 50 years ahead of his time.

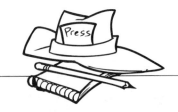

Pilates Scoop

My certification program began around three years ago: two weekend Mat certifications and a 10-week pre-certification to prepare me for the 6-month comprehensive certification program. And I am still learning-and proud of it!

When researching, ask a potential teacher or the studio owner who he studied under. If the teacher is legit, he won't have a problem sharing this information with you. Even today, as the industry exponentially grows, great teachers are often recognized in the industry or your own community. People do talk!

Back then, an apprenticeship provided master teachers an opportunity to live and breathe for Joseph's cause. Many of the master teachers trained for years under Joseph and Clara's supervision. Current demand for teachers, however, is now greater than the supply. As in the good old days, apprenticeships are not practical.

Teachers today are learning the exercises by way of certification. Some programs take a couple years; others are the one-weekend watered-down type. The important point here is not to learn from a teacher who is not certified. This discipline is a specialty form of fitness; it takes months to understand the concepts and to teach you so that you don't get injured.

So, as a future teacher, ask yourself whether you will dedicate a lot of time and spend a lot of money to get certified. As the client, ask yourself whether you are willing to spend more money for a qualified teacher. A reputable certification is demanding and expensive.

If a teacher is dedicated to learning the method, then she won't waste her money on quick fixes. You can't learn Pilates in a weekend. This is not only true for Pilates, but for any profession as well.

To be professional, you must seek out a way to complete your goals. In most cases, that means time, dedication, money, and maybe a little groveling. Learning doesn't stop after you're certified. In fact, it's only the beginning.

Will the Real Pilates Stand Up?

All Pilates is not created a equal! Is it Pilates-based or based on Pilates? Pilates-evolved or evolved from Pilates? Maybe it's the "only," the "true," or the "real" one. Not to mention, Felden-lates! Or Alexander-lates, or Yoga-lates. Will the real Pilates please stand up?

Just like yoga has many styles, Pilates is also developing a repertoire of cross-breeds plus programs that uphold the notion that they are the "only true" Pilates. What's interesting is that Joseph Pilates created this movement by combining Eastern and Western exercise, including yoga. Zen, ancient Grecian regimens, and Roman regimens formed the foundation of his program. Joseph himself adapted his exercises to his clients. In other words, he kept evolving his methods; they were never static. Still, a few of the original master teachers teach their own form of Pilates.

Is that so bad? Not at all. Again, what you teach or want to learn depends on your goals. The beauty of the original work, though, is that it works for many people. The more we learn about how the body moves or is supposed to move, the more timely the Pilates method becomes.

So, when you comb the Yellow Pages or surf the Web, keep in mind that there's no such thing as a "true" Pilates. If so, then Joseph Pilates would be alive and teaching it! If you want to learn or teach the traditional method, then ask the studio owner or teacher what methods are taught. Most studios advertise by advertising "Methods of Joseph Pilates" or the "Teachings of Joseph Pilates."

If they advertise Pilates-based techniques, on the other hand, then maybe they specialize in reconditioning or corrective work. Or, when something is said to be "evolved," does that mean from the original work or evolved from a combination of works?

Many health clubs are combining several body therapies to give their clients more variety, such as yoga-lates. Again, just make sure that the instructors are qualified in their respective fields. After all, how can someone change the original idea if that person doesn't know or understand the concept?

As we move away from fast-paced fitness to slow and controlled movement with the focus on biomechanics, you need to examine the teachers closely. Just don't take it for granted that the gym or health club that you belong to is okay. Check them out because, in the end, it's your body.

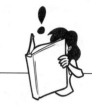

Pilates Primer

Joseph taught different students different variations and techniques, depending on their needs. Pilates is adaptable to the individual, plus it also is capable of improvement that comes with experience and an increase in the knowledge of the human body. It keeps evolving as we do.

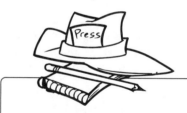

Pilates Scoop

What's amazing about the original Pilates work is that it works for many people. The more we learn about how the body moves or is supposed to move, the more timely the Pilates method becomes.

I've been working in health clubs long enough to know that class sizes can get out of control, meaning 20 students to 1 teacher. There's no way for a qualified teacher to get to every student. If this is the case in your health club, then buy a book or a video, or ask the teacher after class to help you. A good teacher will stay a few minutes after class to address your concerns.

Keep in mind that quasi-exercises are not part of the original method, so they might not be as effective. The original work was designed to do the exercises in order and to follow the prescribed repetitions so that the body develops uniformly. You might not reap the full benefits of the method if exercises are mixed up.

Sign Me Up to Join the Movement

So how long will it take you to learn the exercises, the principles, teaching techniques, and to feel it in your body? Today, time frames vary just as certifications do. Some certifications require anywhere from 275 to 600 hours done over several long and tiresome weekends, and some require internships. The price tag can run $395 to $3,000, excluding private lessons and learning materials.

Some certifications require the potential teacher to have prior experience, such as three to six months of taking private sessions and Mat classes prior to entry. Still others require a practical and written examination along with experience.

Right now, there's not a national registry or national governing body to set standards or guidelines for the Pilates community. All studios and certification programs are self-monitoring. As the method grows, more certifications will be popping up as well.

So what can a hopeful teacher do? How about the likely clients who might not understand what they're getting or even want? As a client searching for a certified instructor, know that the requirements are often demanding. Consider these recommendations for finding a teacher and/or studio:

➤ **Start small.** Attend a Mat class, and hire a teacher to take you through the machines.

➤ **Ask about qualifications.** Are the teachers certified? Where did they get their training?

➤ **Go for quality.** It's very important that you search for quality. With the demand going mainstream, some instructors are getting certified in a weekend. Don't settle for a watered-down version of Joseph's work; it will make a difference in your body.

➤ **Beware of phony claims.** These exercises are not the cure-all. Yes, the exercises are nonimpact and typically are safe for the general population, but that doesn't mean that they will cure you of the common cold if you don't eat right or get plenty of sleep.

➤ **Talk to the teachers.** This is especially true if you have an existing health condition. That way, you can determine for yourself if they're qualified to help you.

➤ **Listen to the rumors.** Teachers talk; we all know how nosy we can be, and most will want to share their stories with you.

➤ **Equipment check.** What kind of equipment does the gym have?

➤ **Check it out.** See if you can come to the teacher's studio to observe.

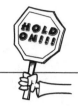

Pilates Precaution

Stay away from programs that claim that they are the "only" real Pilates. Joseph Pilates passed his method on to a handful of master teachers, and then they passed it on, and so forth.

Study the Universal Method

When searching for a certification, you're confronted by dozens of choices. If you're lucky, there will be a studio in your city or nearby that offers some kind of certification. If not, base your decision on what city you would like to spend a lot of time in. Maybe you'll have friends or relatives that you can stay with. Maybe it's driving distance, or you can buy several super-saver tickets. The point is, you will probably spend a good amount of time in that city, so make it as cost-effective and convenient as possible.

After that, give the studio a call. Here's a list of questions that may come in handy:

➤ Do I get certified in both Mat and private instructions?

➤ Can I just get certified in Mat?

➤ What machines do I get certified on?

➤ Is this traditional or a crossbreed of movement?

➤ Can I observe the teachers and your studio?

➤ Will I be able to teach in your studio for internship hours?

➤ Is this vocabulary the traditional vocabulary?

➤ Can I observe a portion of your instructor training session or pay to observe?

➤ Do you have graduates and references that I can speak to?

➤ Is this training reconditioning-based?

➤ Where can I work after I receive your certification?

➤ Is this transferable to other studios and cities?

➤ Will I have a complete understanding of all exercises?

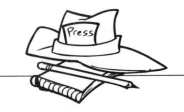

Pilates Scoop

You don't have to be a dancer to make a good teacher. Anyone with compassion, patience, drive, and the intelligence to learn can be a great teacher.

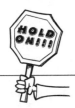

Pilates Precaution

Watch out for certifications that make you pay to use their name. That's like you paying to go to law school, and then you have to pay the institution to say that you graduated from that school—even though you paid to attend in the first place.

➤ Are the exercises demonstrated?

➤ Who will be teaching me, and how long have they been teaching?

➤ How will I learn the exercise? Is it hands-on?

In most programs, you can complete a course in just the Mat. This course usually takes over your entire weekend: Friday night and all day Saturday and Sunday. But don't expect to finish with being able to teach it. You probably won't fully understand or be able to execute all the exercises. You will have to take Mat classes before or after this to fully develop your teaching skills.

On the other hand, no program just teaches the machines. You will always get some Mat work. Some certifications do combine the Mat and machines. To help further, here's a list that roughly defines the training course levels:

➤ **Level I.** The very basic level requires about 15 to 150 hours, with no internship required prior to entry. In most cases, this course is an introduction into the method or Mat certification. Depending on your professional background, this course or certification may improve your teaching skills for other forms of fitness: one-on-one training, aerobics, or yoga. If you do not have an exercise or wellness background, then this information may be overwhelming yet informative. This little amount of time will not certify you in the method.

➤ **Level II.** Certifications under this category require between 150 and 250 hours, with internship requirements. They may or may not require written and practical examinations. This may be a certification on Mat or a precertification to the machines to see if you like it before you plop down a good chunk of money. Typically, there are no prerequisites.

➤ **Level III.** Programs under this category require between 275 and 375 hours, with internship and continuing education requirements. Written and practical examinations are administered. At this level, you may learn to teach the basic beginner exercises on the equipment, plus get lectures in anatomy. There's usually a prerequisite of 10 to 30 hours of lessons or workshops or anatomy seminars.

➤ **Level IV.** Programs under this category require 400 to 600 hours, plus internships and continuing education. Written and practical examinations are given to complete the certification. At this level, you'll complete the full spectrum of equipment and Mat, plus maybe get some ideas on exercises that recondition the body. Requirements of 60 or more lessons may or may not have an entrance examination or a practical screening prior to acceptance into program.

Avoid the Quacks

There's not a particular time limit on how or when you will be certified or allowed to teach on your own. That depends on you and how well your mind and body absorb the information. For example, learning the Mat exercises, which is least demanding, usually takes an entire weekend of training, plus six months or more of taking other Mat classes, plus follow-up training.

Or, you may have a background in dance, so you pick up the Mat concepts in a couple weeks. There's no telling when you'll learn the 500 exercises, core concepts, and program designs.

The primary problem with this industry is that there's no standardization. Here are some tips to help you distinguish between the knowledgeable instructors and the quacks:

➤ Avoid certifications that espouse a one-weekend certification.

➤ Avoid certifications that advocate their way as the only way.

➤ Avoid certifications that make you pay for using their name.

➤ Avoid certifications that make you sign a long-term contract.

➤ Avoid certifications that disparage other certifications, the medical community, chiropractors, or physical therapists.

Pilates Scoop

If you want to get certified on the Mat and equipment, the money and time commitment is huge. It takes about one to two years to complete all the requirements and to take private sessions. Certification also costs (by the time it's all done) $5,000 to $8,000.

The Universal Method Is Here for Good!

Unlike other forms of fitness, the more we learn about how the body works, the more appropriate the Pilates method is. Life goes in a never-ending circle. What was once old is now new and, in some weird way, connected.

Here we are, in a new millennium, and the universal method zooms the globe. Yet follow its roots and you could argue that Pilates started in India in the sixth century by monks practicing yoga, or in ancient Greece in the athletic era when men dazzled audiences as they performed physical feats in the Olympics.

We're paying tribute to a man who invented a sophisticated method that began in ancient times and will no doubt endure the sands of time. Thanks to the devoted master teachers who spread the word and kept the Pilates work alive, we have it today. The truth is, these teachers taught Pilates when it wasn't fashionable. The financial returns were not great. So why did they do it? Probably because they believed in the ideal fitness and the man who invented it, Joseph Pilates. Probably because they witnessed firsthand how this method can change the body and mind for the better. Probably because they loved it!

As research continues to multiply and contradict itself, people will search for a new way to work the body. There's no contradictory research for this method. As we get older, we don't want to climb the Stairmaster or limp through an aerobics class, or lift endless reps. You no longer have to be the one-set wonder, aerobics queen, or king of the treadmill. There are plenty of exercises ranging in degree of difficulty and variety that will keep you challenged and aging gracefully.

A Growing Trend

It's only a matter of time before overuse injuries plaque the fitness industry because of a lack of moderation—myself included! I was and still am an integral part of the aerobics evolution; I still teach all that jazzy choreography, only not eight classes a week. The Pilates ideologies changed the way I work out. I think about my movement and now listen to my body. I have more strength now, even though fitness has always been part of my life. Don't get me wrong—I still enjoy a great sweat, but I now know that there's something better to develop my mind and define my body.

Maybe that will happen to you, too. Perhaps the Pilates vision of the ideal fitness is catching on. No longer will it be kept a secret among on elite athletes and celebrities. As the movement grows, it can be yours.

Fitness clubs and gyms are building small studios and hiring personal trainers. Mat classes are now common on the weekly class schedule. And why? Because, in the end, we want better bodies and a workout that leaves us feeling great about ourselves. This, then, is your ideal fitness; you see it, feel it, and have it!

"The Prophecy: In 10 sessions, you'll feel the difference; in 20, you'll see the difference; and in 30, you'll have a whole new body." Words to live by, from Joseph Pilates.

The Least You Need to Know

➤ For years, master teachers have passed on Joseph Pilates's work.

➤ Teachers today are learning the exercises by way of certification, which can take a year to two years to complete.

➤ Future teachers should ask themselves whether they can dedicate a lot of time and spend a lot of money to get certified.

➤ Clients should ask themselves whether they are willing to spend more money for a qualified teacher.

➤ Unlike other forms of fitness, the more we learn about how the body works, the more appropriate the Pilates method is.

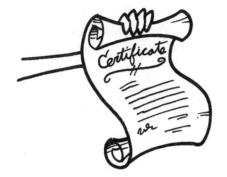

Certification Programs

So you want to join the team that makes up the Pilates world. Here's a list of contacts.

Teacher Certifications

Core Dynamics
P.O. Box 22983
Santa Fe, NM 87502
Phone 505-988-5076
Contact: Michele Lawson (founder)

Physicalmind Institute
1807 Second Street, Suite 40
Santa Fe, NM 87505
Phone 800-505-1990
Web site: www.methodfitness.com

Polestar Education, LLC
1500 Monza Ave., Suite 350
Coral Gables, FL 33146
Phone 1-800-387-3651 or 305-666-0037
Fax 305-666-1808
E-mail: info@polestareducation.com
Web site: www.polestareducation.com
Contact: Elizabeth Larkham or Brent Anderson (co-founders)

Stott Pilates International Certification Center
2200 Yonge St., Suite 1402
Toronto, CA M4S 2C6
Phone 416-482-4050
Fax 416-482-2742
Web site: www.stottconditioning.com

The Pilates Studio
2121 Broadway
New York, New York 10023
Phone 212-875-0189
Web site: www.pilates-studio.com

The Pilates Center of Austin
5555 North LaMar Blvd., Suite E103
Austin, TX 78751
Phone 512-467-8009
Web site: www.pilates@pilatescenterofaustin.com

The Pilates Center Boulder
4800 Base Line Road
Boulder, CO 80303
Phone 303-494-3400
Web site: www.thepilatescenter.com

The Pilates Method Alliance
Phone 877-528-3335
Web site: www.pilatesmethodalliance.org
Contact: Kevin Bowen/Colleen Glenn

The System Certification Program
Goodbodys
5301 West Lovers Lane
Suite 114
Dallas, Texas 75209
Phone 877-528-3335
Web site: www.goodbodys.com
Contact: Colleen Glenn

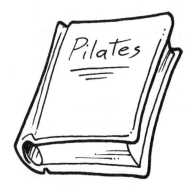

Glossary

This appendix contains words or common lingo used in Pilates—some words that Joseph Pilates conjured up himself! Lengthen your lingo, and you're on your way to learning Pilates. Good luck.

aerobic   Exercises that use oxygen, such as running, walking, and so on.

anaerobic   Exercises that don't use oxygen, such as weight training, sprinting, and so on.

atrophy   The state when the muscles waste away to the point at which you can't engage in day-to-day activities. This doesn't happen because of old age, but because of an inactive, sedentary lifestyle.

bone by bone   Phrase that refers to the act of stacking your vertebra one at a time. This core concept is used in almost every exercise, so get used to peeling your spine up and down.

bone in its joint   Phrase that refers to the joint is in its proper place. This proper joint alignment permits the limbs to move safely in a wide variety of movements without wear and tear on the joint. *Bone in its joint* particularly pertains to the ball-and-socket joints of the hips and shoulder joints. Remember, first you stabilize the body, and then you move it!

business plan   A blueprint of how you plan to grow your gym. It will tell your future investors what you're going to do, how you're going to do it, and the time frame you'll do it in.

chin to your chest   The safest position for your head, neck, and back; it works in line with gravity to hold your head in a safe position.

concentric contraction   Contraction that shortens the muscle.

cross-training   Method of building overall fitness with multiple activities. Complete fitness usually cannot be achieved with just one single sport, so cross-training is a must to prevent injury, burnout, and overtraining, whether it's mental or physical.

diaphragm   Partition of muscles and tendons in the midriff. When you draw air in, your diaphragm relaxes and moves downward to create a vacuum, sort of like pushing an accordion in and out to generate music. This vacuum draws air into the lungs. To get rid of the air, the diaphragm contracts and rises up to push all the air out of your lungs.

eccentric contraction   Contraction that lengthens the muscle.

Grand Ronde de Jambe   Exercise whose name, in French, actually means "big leg circles."

isometric contraction   Contraction in which the muscle doesn't move when it's contracted.

kyphosis posture   An exaggerated curve in the thoracic spine, your upper back.

lengthen   The action of "growing yourself tall." This length comes from the spine, as if you're pulled up from the top of your head by a string.

levator scapulae   One of the major neck muscles, which starts just below the back of the skull and ends at the scapula.

lordosis   An exaggeration of the curvature to the lumber region.

metabolism   How the body burns calories. You can be doing absolutely nothing, and your body will burn calories. You can alter your metabolic rate by increasing your lean muscle mass and reducing your overall fat.

movement muscles   Muscles that tend to be superficial in nature.

neutral pelvis   Position in which the spine is in its natural length. To find neutral pelvis on your body, feel the little bony protrusions toward the top of the pelvis, known as the iliac crests. With the heel of your hand, feel your pubic bone. Find the distance between those two points, and lay your hand flat.

peeling your spine off   Action of rolling your back off the Mat as if picking up a string of pearls one at a time. The Mat or spinal articulation protects the back as you roll up and down, increases the flexibility of the spine, and works the powerhouse.

Pilates box   Term meaning to work within the boundaries of your torso, no wider than your shoulders and hips.

Pilates stance   Stance in which the feet are slightly turned out from the heels so that you make a small "V." The feet are no wider than three fingers apart.

pinch your butt cheeks   Posture in which you imagine a thousand-dollar bill between your butt cheeks and then squeeze to work all the right areas: the butt cheeks, the upper back of the inner thighs, and the ever-so-vital pelvic floor muscles that keep your internal organs and muscles from dropping out of your body.

pinch, lift, and grow   The length that comes from your spine as the head floats up, lifting every bone. Pinch your butt cheeks so that you grow even taller. This position is a neutral pelvis, meaning that the pelvis does not tilt.

powerhouse Your muscular girdle of strength. The powerhouse sort of looks like a thick rubber band or corset that wraps around the middle part of your body; it expands from the bottom of your rib cage to the line across your hips and wraps around to your back.

pronation Position in which you turn in your ankles so that the body weight is unnaturally displaced on the arches of your feet.

proprioceptive system Literally, "own reception." Proprioception coordinates every movement in time and space.

push from the tush Action in which you initiate the movement from your bottom: your tush, upper thighs, the back of the upper thighs, and your powerhouse.

scapula stabilization Action in which you pull the shoulders slightly back and then down, as if your shoulder blades are drawing down your back. Think of the muscles underneath your arms preparing you for the movement—your pits to your hips.

self-talk Thinking or talking to yourself—a type of internal communication; use this mental training method to enhance physical performance.

serratus anterior A broad, thin muscle covering the lateral rib cage and connecting to your shoulder blades. It holds your shoulder blades in place, which helps to stabilize your shoulders.

shoulder girdle The main purpose of the shoulder girdle is to connect the arms to the body. This structure is stabilized by a group of muscles called the rotator cuff, or shoulder rotators, for short. The *subscapularis, supraspinatus, infraspinatus,* and *teres minor* encircle the shoulder joint so that the large movement muscles can move with ease.

Spine Corrector Sometimes called the Small Barrel is a light-weight padded apparatus that looks like a small barrel and is used to work the abdominals and correct posture; it's safe enough for anyone to use, from pregnant moms to the octogenarian, to the client with posture issues.

spine to Mat, or anchor your spine Position in which you imagine that your torso weighs 50 pounds; it's heavy and is anchored to the floor.

stabilizing muscles Deep muscles hidden between, under, and behind some of the more common muscles. The transverse is a perfect example of a stabilizing muscle.

sternocleidomastoid A major neck muscle that attaches to two bones in the front of your body: the breast bone and the clavicle.

supination Action in which you roll out the ankles, which could negatively affect the muscle tone and shape of the leg from the ankles to the hips.

synovial fluids The body's natural version of WD-40 for your joints. When you move, especially in a slow, controlled manner, you're increasing synovial fluid production, whether it's in the spine, hip, shoulder, or other part of the body. This keeps your joints flexible, protects them from seizing up, and perhaps prevents one of today's most debilitating disease—arthritis.

theory of opposition   This theory moves the body in two different directions to engage more muscle groups; it increases the resistance of all the exercises and gets you in touch with your body.

transversus abdominis   The deepest of abdominal muscles, sometimes called the Transverse.

upper trapezius   A major neck muscle that runs from the base of the skull past the scapula.

visualization   The act of strengthening your inner power so that you can achieve the results you want. Train the brain, and your body will physically respond.

Index

A

abdominal muscles
  oblique muscles, 29
  results of crunches/sit-ups, 89
  securing your scoop, 90
  transversus abdominis muscle, 29
advanced exercises
  Advanced Teaser (adding intensity to Teaser 1), 128
  Bicycle, 141
  Boomerang, 147-149
  Can-Can, 141-142
  Double-Leg Kick, 109
  Fives Series, 106
    Crisscross, 108
    Double Straight-Leg Stretch, 107
    Straight-Leg Stretch, 106
  Hip Circles, 142-143
  Jackknife, 126-127
  Kneeling Side Kicks, 144
  Leg Pull Back, 115, 130
  Leg Pull Front, 113-114, 129
  Mermaid, 145
  Push-Ups, 130-131
  Rollover, 122-123
  Scissors, 140
  Shoulder Bridge, 110-111
    adding intensity with kicks, 124-125
  Spine Twist, 125-126
  Swan Dive (adding intensity to the Swan), 138
  Swimming, 112-113
  Teaser 1, 111-112
  Twist, 145, 147
Advanced Teaser exercise (adding intensity to Teaser 1), 128
aerobic production of energy, 38
aging, 10
aligning your body, posture, 30
anaerobic production of energy, 38
anatomy of the spine, 21-22
  discs, 21
  spinal cord, 21
  vertebrae, 21
Anchor your Spine (Spine to Mat), 64

Ankle Circles exercise, 79
anticellulite solution, sculpting your bottom half, 151
  Side Kick Series, 152-164
arch of back, *lordosis* posture, 25
Arm Circles
  exercise, 174-175
    Barrels, 229
  Reformer Stomach Massage Series, 192
arms
  exercises
    Leaning into the Wind, 168
    Standing Arm Series, 169-177
  muscles
    biceps, 168
    triceps, 168
Arms Back, Reformer Stomach Massage Series, 191
art of teaching, 246
  commitment, 246, 254
  dancers, 253-254
  dealing with clients, 251
    developing step-by-step progression, 251-252
    hands-on training, 252
    patience, 253
    practicing KISS, 252
    praising results, 253
  designing custom programs, FIT (Frequency, Intensity, and Time), 248-251
  desire, 256
  emotional support system, 247
  getting to know students, 247-248
  listening to clients, 255
  strategies for the teacher, 249
  treatment of clients, 254
assessing body changes, 51-52
athletic performance, 14
  holistic training, 14-15
  muscle strength and length, 15-16
atrophy, 10
auxiliary equipment, Cadillac, 198
Ayurveda (Indian healing art), 35

B

back
  arch, *lordosis* posture, 25
  muscles
    latissimus dorsi, 168
    rhomboids, 168
    serratus anterior, 168
    trapezius, 168
Backward Stretch exercise (Barrels), 225
balance
  Open-Leg Rocker exercise, 93-94
  Wunda Chair, 211-212
    challenge, 213
    cost, 212
    functions, 212
    Jackknife exercise, 217
    Pike exercise, 214
    safety, 213
    sequence of exercises, 213
    Spine Stretch exercise, 218
    springs, 213
    Stretch with Pumping Arms exercise, 216
    Swan exercise, 216-217
    Washer Woman exercise, 214
Barrels (equipment), 221-228
  exercises, 223-226
    Arm Circles, 229
    Backward Stretch, 225
    Bicycle, 227-228
    Horseback, 224
    Low Barrel, 226
    Rolling In and Out, 228
    Scissors, 227
    sequence, 224
  functions, 223
  Ladder Barrel, cost, 221-222
  Spine Corrector, cost, 222
Beat-Beat Up exercise, as part of Side Kick Series, 155
Beats on the Belly exercise, as part of Side Kick Series, 156
beginner exercises, 73-74
  Ankle Circles, 79
  Double-Leg Stretch, 83
  Hamstring Stretch, 78-79
  Hundred, 75-76
  Leg Circles, 79-80

Roll-Up, 77
Rolling Like a Ball, 80
  wobble-free rolls, 81
Saw, 84-85
Seal, 86
Single-Leg Stretch, 82
Spine Stretch, 84
"V" stance, 74-75
Beginner Work (weeks 1 and 2),
  52
Beginner-Intermediate Work
  (weeks 3 and 4), 52
benefits
  Pilates Method, 17-18
  Reformer, 182-183
Biceps Curls exercise, 170
biceps muscles, 168
Bicycle exercise, 141
  as part of Side Kick Series,
    163-164
  Barrels, 227-228
  Cadillac Leg Spring Series,
    206
Big O. *See* Magic Circle
Birds' Feet, Footwork Series
  (Reformer), 187
body
  awareness of form, 61
  connection to mind, 135
    breathing control,
      136-138
    imagery, 135-138
  conscious versus uncon-
    scious movement, 60-61
  movement muscles, *rectus
    femoris*, 58
  muscle imbalances, training
    with symmetry, 59
  stabilizing muscles, *trans-
    versus abdominal*, 58
  therapy, 6-7
  working from within,
    stabilizing muscles
bone by bone movement (vertebrae), 22
bone care
  calcium, 11
  collagen, 11
  osteoporosis prevention,
    11-12
bone in its joint, 79
booking clients, teaching as a
  business, 263
Boomerang exercise, 147-149
Boxing exercise, 171
breathing, 33
  aerobic production of
    energy, 38
  anaerobic production of
    energy, 38

Cadillac, 201-202
controlled (training guiding
  principle), 48
deep breaths, 36
detoxifying your body,
  37-38
  Spine Twist exercise,
    125-126
diaphragmatic, 35
enhancing overall health,
  33-34
increasing stamina, 39
mind and body connection,
  136-138
practicing, 40-41
process, 35-37
rules, 41
  avoid holding breath, 42
  avoid running on empty,
    42
  monitor breathing,
    43-44
  stop mouth-breathing, 43
  vow to get more air,
    42-43
  versus respirations, 35-36
breathometer, 41
business of teaching
  attracting investors with a
    business plan, 260-261
  booking clients, 263
  choosing location, 265
  determining space needed,
    264-265
  equipment costs, 258
  figuring potential profits,
    263
  hiring teachers, 263
  homebody versus gym body,
    257-258
  legalities, 258-260
  marketing, 265-266
  purchasing equipment,
    266-267
butt, anticellulite solution, 151
  Side Kick Series, 152-164

C

Cadillac (equipment), 197
  as auxiliary equipment, 198
  cost, 198
  exercises, 200
    breathing, 201-202
    Half-Hang, 208
    Hanging Up, 208
    Leg Spring Series,
      203-206
    Monkey, 207

Rolling Back, 201
  sequence, 200
  functions, 199
  safety rules, 199-200
  trapeze, 198
calcium, 11
Can-Can exercise, 141-142
centering (training guiding
  principle), 47
cerebral cortex, 60
certifications
  course levels, 274
    Level I, 274
    Level II, 274
    Level III, 274
    Level IV, 275
  lack of standardization, 275
  programs, 279
    searching, 273-275
  time commitment, 272-273
cervical vertebrae, 23
chest muscles
  pectoralis major, 168
  pectoralis minor, 168
Chest Expansion exercise, 175
Child's Pose (relaxation position), 99
Chin to your Chest exercise, 67
cilia, 43
cleaning equipment, 266-267
clients
  strategies for teachers, 251
    developing step-by-step
      progression, 251-252
    hands-on training, 252
    patience, 253
    practicing KISS, 252
    praise results, 253
    teaching, booking in your
      business, 263
Close the Hatch exercise, as
  part of Side Kick Series, 159
coccygeal vertebrae, 23
collagen, 11
commitment
  obtaining certification,
    272-273
  teaching, 246, 254
compatibility of Pilates with
  other fitness programs, 51
concentration (training guiding
  principle), 46
concentric contraction, 91
concepts
  core, 71
    Chin to your Chest, 67
    Just for Feet, 71
    Peel your Spine Off the
      Mat, 64-65
    Pelvic Clocks, 66

Pinch your Butt Cheeks, 70
Pinch, Lift, and Grow Tall, 70-71
Pits to your Hips, 68-69
Pregnant Cat, 63
Scoop, 62-63
Spine to Mat, 64
exercises, 61-62
conscious movement versus unconscious, 60-61
contraction of muscles, 91
concentric, 91
eccentric, 91
isometric, 91
control (training guiding principle), 46, 92
Contrology, 5
coordination, Single-Leg Kick exercise, 97-98
core fitness, cross-training, 17
Corkscrew exercise, 94-95
costs
Barrels
Ladder Barrel, 222
Spine Corrector, 222
Cadillac, 198
equipment, 258
Magic Circle, 232
Universal Reformer, 182
Wunda Chair, 212
course levels (training), 274
Level I, 274
Level II, 274
Level III, 274
Level IV, 275
Crisscross exercise, as part of Fives Series, 108
cross-training, 17
crunches, 89
securing your scoop, 90
curves of the spine, 23
custom programs, FIT (Frequency, Intensity, and Time), 248
Frequency, 249-250
Intensity, 250
Time, 251

D

dancers, teaching Pilates, 253-254
deep breaths, 36
deltoid muscles, 168
Fly exercise, 172-173
Zip-Up exercise, 173

designing custom programs, FIT (Frequency, Intensity, and Time), 248
Frequency, 249-250
Intensity, 250
Time, 251
detoxifying your body, breathing, 37-38
Spine Twist exercise, 125-126
developing step-by-step progression (teaching), 251-252
diaphragm, 36-37
diaphragmatic breathing, 35
discs (spine), 21
Double Straight-Leg Stretch, as part of Fives Series, 107
Double-Leg Kick exercise, 109
Double-Leg Lift exercise, as part of Side Kick Series, 158
Double-Leg Stretch exercise, 83
dowager's hump, 11

E

eating, thermogenesis, 49
eccentric contraction, 91
Electric Chair. *See* High Chair
emotional support system, teaching, 247
endorphins, 39
endurance. *See* stamina
energy
aerobic production, 38
anaerobic production, 38
equipment
Barrels, 221-229
Arm Circles exercise, 229
Backward Stretch exercise, 225
Bicycle exercise, 227-228
functions, 223
Horseback exercise, 224
Ladder Barrel, 221-222
Low Barrel exercises, 226
Rolling In and Out exercise, 228
Scissors exercise, 227
sequence of exercises, 224
Spine Corrector, 222
Cadillac, 197-200
as auxiliary equipment, 198
breathing, 201-202
cost, 198
functions, 199
Half-Hang, 208
Hanging Up, 208
Leg Spring Series, 203-206

Monkey, 207
Rolling Back, 201
safety rules, 199-200
sequence, 200
trapeze, 198
cleaning, 266-267
costs, 258
High Chair, 212
Magic Circle, 231-232
cost, 232
functions, 232
Hundred exercise, 233
Leg Work, 235-237
Pelvic Lifts exercise, 233-234
sequence of exercises, 232-233
Standing Arm Work, 234
Wall Work, 237-241
purchasing for your business, 266-267
Universal Reformer, 181-195
benefits, 182-183
cost, 182
foot work, 183-185
Footwork Series, 186-188
Hundred, 188-189
Knee Stretches, 194-195
Leg Circles, 190
Running, 195
sequence of exercises, 185-186
Short Box Series, 192-194
springs, 182
Stomach Massage Series, 190-192
Wunda Chair, 211-217
challenge, 213
cost, 212
functions, 212
Jackknife exercise, 217
Pike exercise, 214
safety, 213
sequence of exercises, 213
Spine Stretch exercise, 218
springs, 213
Stretch with Pumping Arms exercise, 216
Swan exercise, 216-217
Washer Woman exercise, 214
exercises
advanced
Advanced Teaser, 128
Bicycle, 141
Boomerang, 147, 149
Can-Can, 141-142

Double-Leg Kick, 109
Fives Series, 106-108
Hip Circles, 142-143
Jackknife, 126-127
Kneeling Side Kicks, 144
Leg Pull Back, 115, 130
Leg Pull Front, 113-114, 129
Mermaid, 145
Push-Ups, 130-131
Rollover, 122-123
Scissors, 140
Shoulder Bridge, 110-111, 124-125
Spine Twist, 125-126
Swan Dive, 138
Swimming, 112-113
Teaser 1, 111-112
Twist, 145, 147
arms
    Leaning into the Wind, 168
    Standing Arm Series, 169-177
Barrels, 224-229
    Arm Circles, 229
    Backward Stretch, 225
    Bicycle, 227-228
    Horseback, 224
    Low Barrel, 226
    Rolling In and Out, 228
    Scissors, 227
beginners, 73-74
    Ankle Circles, 79
    Double-Leg Stretch, 83
    Hamstring Stretch, 78-79
    Hundred, 75-76
    Leg Circles, 79-80
    Roll-Up, 77
    Rolling Like a Ball, 80-81
    Saw, 84-85
    Seal, 86
    Single-Leg Stretch, 82
    Spine Stretch, 84
    "V" stance, 74-75
Cadillac, 200
    breathing, 201-202
    Half-Hang, 208
    Hanging Up, 208
    Leg Spring Series, 203-206
    Monkey, 207
    Rolling Back, 201
    sequence, 200
core concepts, 71
    Chin to your Chest, 67
    Just for Feet, 71

Peel your Spine Off the Mat, 64-65
Pelvic Clocks, 66
Pinch your Butt Cheeks, 70
Pinch, Lift, and Grow Tall, 70-71
Pits to your Hips, 68-69
Pregnant Cat, 63
Scoop, 62-63
Spine to Mat, 64
intermediate, 92
    Child's Pose, 99
    Corkscrew, 94-95
    Neck Pull, 99-100
    Open-Leg Rocker, 93-94
    Single-Leg Kick, 97-98
    Swan, 95-97
learning concepts, language of Pilates, 61-62
Magic Circle
    Hundred, 233
    Leg Work, 235-237
    Pelvic Lifts, 233-234
    sequence, 232-233
    Standing Arm Work, 234
    Wall Work, 237-241
rhythm, 104
Universal Reformer, 185
    Footwork Series, 186-188
    Hundred, 188-189
    Knee Stretches, 194-195
    Leg Circles, 190
    Running, 195
    sequence, 185-186
    Short Box Series, 192-194
    Stomach Massage Series, 190-192
Wunda Chair
    Jackknife exercise, 217
    Pike exercise, 214
    sequence, 213
    Spine Stretch exercise, 218
    Stretch with Pumping Arms exercise, 216
    Swan exercise, 216-217
    Washer Woman exercise, 214
external intercostal muscles, 36

F

feet, Reformer, 183-185
Fists in the Belly exercise, Reformer Short Box Series, 192

FIT (Frequency, Intensity, and Time), 249
    Frequency, 249-250
    Intensity, 250
    Time, 251
fitness
    assessing body changes, 51-52
    building up your body, 45-46
    dividing weeks to get started, 52
        Beginner Work (weeks 1 and 2), 52
        Beginner-Intermediate Work (weeks 3 and 4), 52
        Intermediate Work (weeks 5 and 6), 52
    metabolism, 48
        thermogenesis, 49
    Pilates compatibility with other programs, 51
    training, 46
        guiding principles, 46-48, 92, 103
        plans, 50
Fives Series, 106
    Crisscross, 108
    Double Straight-Leg Stretch, 107
    Straight-Leg Stretch, 106
Flat Back exercise, Reformer Short Box Series, 193
flexibility of the spine, Rollover exercise, 122-123
flow, maintaining (training guiding principle), 47, 103
Flutter Kicks exercise, as part of Side Kick Series, 160
Fly exercise, 172-173
Footwork Series (Universal Reformer), 186-188
    Birds' Feet, 187
    Heels, 187
    Tendon Stretch, 187
    "V", 187
form, awareness when performing exercises, 61
Frequency (part of FIT), 249-250
Frequency, Intensity, and Time. *See* FIT
Frog exercise (Cadillac), Leg Spring Series, 205
functions (equipment)
    Barrels, 223
    Cadillac, 199
    Magic Circle, 232
    Wunda Chair, 212

G

girdle of strength. *See* power-house
Grande Ronde de Jambe exercise, as part of Side Kick Series, 161-162
grow yourself tall. *See* lengthening
guiding principles (training), 46
  centering, 47
  concentration, 46
  control, 46, 92
  controlled breathing, 48
  maintaining flow, 47, 103
  precision, 47
Gut Buster exercises (Magic Circle)
  Hundred, 233
  Pelvic Lifts, 233-234
gymnasium
  equipment costs, 258
  versus homebody, 257-258

H

Half-Hang exercise (Cadillac), 208
Hamstring Stretch exercise, 78-79
hands-on training (teaching), 252
Hanging Up exercise (Cadillac), 208
happy joint, 77
head, positioning in slumping posture, 25
Heel Beats exercise (Cadillac), Leg Spring Series, 204-205
Heels, Footwork Series (Reformer), 187
High Chair, 212
Hip Circles exercise, 142-143
hip stabilization, 70
hiring teachers, teaching as a business, 263
history of instruction, 269-270
holding breath, 42
holistic training, athletic performance, 14-15
homebody
  equipment costs, 258
  versus gym body, 257-258
Horseback exercise (Barrels), 224
Hot Potato exercise, as part of Side Kick Series, 161

Hundred, 75-76
  Magic Circle, 233
  Universal Reformer, 188-189

I

illiopsoas muscle, 90
imagery, mind and body connection, 135-138
imbalances of muscles, correction with Pilates, 16
increasing stamina with breathing, 39
individual instruction, 8-9
infraspinatus rotator cuff muscle, 168
Inner Thigh Circles exercise, as part of Side Kick Series, 159
integration of muscle groups, 105
intensity
  as part of FIT, 250
  increasing
    Advanced Teaser exercise, 128
    Leg Pull Back exercise, 130
    Leg Pull Front exercise, 129
    Shoulder Bridge exercise, 124-125
    Swan Dive exercise, 138
intercostal muscles
  external, 36
  internal, 36
intermediate exercises, 92
  Child's Pose, 99
  Corkscrew, 94-95
  Neck Pull, 99-100
  Open-Leg Rocker, 93-94
  Single-Leg Kick, 97-98
  Swan, 95-97
Intermediate Work (weeks 5 and 6), 52
internal intercostal muscles, 36
investors, teaching as a business, business plan, 260-261
isometric contraction, 91

J–K

Jackknife exercise, 126-127
  Wunda Chair, 217
joints
  bone in its joint, 79
  happy, 77
Just for Feet exercise, 71

Kaiser Institute on Aging, 11
Keep It Simple, Sweetie! (teaching style). *See* KISS
kicks
  adding to Shoulder Bridge exercise, 124-125
  Double-Leg, 109
  Flutter, 160
  Kneeling Side, 144
KISS (Keep It Simple, Sweetie!), teaching style, 252
Knee Stretches (Universal Reformer), 194-195
Kneeling Side Kicks exercise, 144
kyphosis posture, 24

L

lactic acid, 38
  accumulation with over-tensing muscles, 166
Ladder Barrel (Large Barrel equipment), 221
  cost, 222
language of Pilates Method, 62
Large Barrel. *See* Ladder Barrel
latissimus dorsi muscle, 28, 168
Leaning into the Wind exercise, 168
learning exercises
  concepts, 61-62
  language of Pilates, 62
Leg Circles
  Cadillac Leg Spring Series, 203
  exercise, 79-80
  Universal Reformer, 190
Leg Pull Back exercise, 115
  adding intensity, 130
Leg Pull Front exercise, 113-114
  adding intensity, 129
Leg Spring Series (Cadillac), 203
  Bicycle, 206
  Frog, 205
  Heel Beats, 204-205
  Leg Circles, 203
  Marches, 204
Leg Work (Magic Circle), 235-237
legalities, teaching as a business, 258-260
length of muscles, athletic performance, 15-16, 91
lengthening, 27
levator scapulae muscle, 167
Level I course (training course), 274

Level II course (training course), 274

Level III course (training course), 274

Level IV course (training course), 275

listening to clients (teaching), 255

lordosis posture, 25

Low Barrel exercises, 226

Lower-Body Buster exercises (Magic Circle), Leg Work, 235-237

M

Magic Circle (equipment), 231-237
  cost, 232
  exercises
    Hundred, 233
    Leg Work, 235-237
    Pelvic Lifts, 233-234
    sequence, 232-233
    Standing Arm Work, 234
    Wall Work, 237-241
  functions, 232
March exercise (Cadillac), Leg Spring Series, 204
marketing, attracting clients to business, 265-266
Mat workouts, 8-9
memory, ability of muscles, 60
Mermaid exercise, 145
messages communicated by your body, 19
metabolism, 48
  thermogenesis, 49
mind and body connection, 135
  breathing control, 136-138
  imagery, 135-138
mind-breath connection, 35
monitoring breathing, 43-44
Monkey exercise (Cadillac), 207
mouth-breathing, avoiding (breathing rule), 43
movement muscles, *rectus femoris*, 58
muscles
  arms
    biceps, 168
    triceps, 168
  atrophy, 10
  back
    latissimus dorsi, 168
    rhomboids, 168
    serratus anterior, 168
    trapezius, 168

chest
  pectoralis major, 168
  pectoralis minor, 168
conscious versus unconscious movement, 60-61
contraction, 91
  concentric, 91
  eccentric, 91
  isometric, 91
endurance, 105
external intercostals, 36
illiopsoas, 90
imbalances
  correction with Pilates, 16
  training with symmetry, 59
internal intercostals, 36
length, athletic performance, 15-16
lengthening, 91
memory, 60
movement, *rectus femoris*, 58
neck
  aches and stiffness, 167
  levator scapulae, 167
  sternocleidomastoid, 167
  upper trapezius, 167
obliques, 29
overtensing, 166
  accumulation of lactic acid, 166
  upper trapezius, 166
serratus anterior, 68
shoulders, 167
  deltoids, 168
  rotator cuff, 168
spinal support, 28
  latissimus dorsi, 28
  rhomboids, 28
  serratus anterior, 28
  trapezius muscle, 28
stabilizing, *transversus abdominal*, 58
strength, athletic performance, 15-16
transversus abdominis, 29

N–O

Navel to Spine exercise (Scoop), 62-63
neck muscles
  aches and stiffness, 167
  levator scapulae, 167
  sternocleidomastoid, 167
  upper trapezius, 167
Neck Pull exercise, 99-100
neutral pelvis position, 26-27

obliques
  muscles, 29
  Side Stretch exercise, 176
one vertebra at a time movement, 22
Open-Leg Rocker exercise, 93-94
opposition, theory of, 120-121
osteoporosis, prevention with resistance training, 11-12
overtensing the muscles, 166
  accumulation of lactic acid, 166
  upper trapezius, 166
oxygen, 35

P

Parallel Leg exercise, as part of Side Kick Series, 158
patience (teaching), 253
pectoralis major muscle, 168
pectoralis minor muscle, 168
Peel your Spine Off the Mat exercise, 64-65
Pelvic Clocks exercises, 66
Pelvic Lifts exercise (Magic Circle), 233-234
pelvis
  neutral position, 26-27
  Wall Work (Magic Circle), 237-241
physical training, 15
Pike exercise (Wunda Chair), 214
Pilates box, 171
Pilates Method
  aging, 10
  as a rehabilitative program, 9-10
  benefits, 17-18
  body therapy, 6-7
  compatibility with other programs, 51
  correction of muscle imbalances, 16
  history of instruction, 269-270
  individual instruction, 8-9
  language, 62
  Mat workouts, 8-9
  osteoporosis prevention, 11-12
    resistance training, 12
  pregnancy, 12
    practicing pre-pregnancy, 12-13
    safety precautions, 13-14

testimonies, 3-5
thinking body, 5-6
variations in style and instruction, 270-272
Pilates, Joseph (founder of Pilates Method), 3, 7-8
Pinch your Butt Cheeks exercise, 70
Pinch, Lift, and Grow Tall exercise, 70-71
Pits to your Hips exercise, 68-69
posture, 20-21
    anatomy of the spine, 21-22
        discs, 21
        spinal cord, 21
        vertebrae, 21
    arch in back, *lordosis* posture, 25
    curves of the spine, 23
    neutral pelvis position, 26-27
    powerhouse, 29
        oblique muscles, 29
        transversus abdominis muscle, 29
    slumping, 23
        head positioning, 25
        kyphosis, 24
        shoulder positioning, 24-25
    spinal support, 28
        latissimus dorsi, 28
        rhomboids, 28
        serratus anterior, 28
        trapezius muscle, 28
    thinking yourself tall, 30
powerhouse, 29
    oblique muscles, 29
    transversus abdominis muscle, 29
practicing breathing, 40-41
praising results (teaching), 253
precision (training guiding principle), 47
pregnancy, 12
    practicing Pilates pre-pregnancy, 12-13
    safety precautions, 13-14
Pregnant Cat exercise, 63
prevention of osteoporosis, 11-12
    resistance training, 12
process of breathing, 35-37
profits, teaching as a business, 263
programs, certification, 279
progression, developing tool to track, 251-252

pronation, 184
proprioceptive system, 5-6
psoas. See illiopsoas muscle
psychological training, 15
purchasing equipment, business plans, 266-267
push from the tush, 106
Push-Ups exercises, 130-131

R

Rack. *See* Reformer
rectus femoris muscle, 58
Reformer (equipment), 181-195
    benefits, 182-183
    cost, 182
    exercises, 185
        Footwork Series, 186-188
        Hundred, 188-189
        Knee Stretches, 194-195
        Leg Circles, 190
        Running, 195
        sequence, 185-186
        Short Box Series, 192-194
        Stomach Massage Series, 190-192
    foot work, 183-185
    springs, 182
relaxation, Child's Pose, 99
resistance training, osteoporosis prevention, 12
respirations versus breathing, 35-36
respiratory system, 35
rhomboid muscles, 28, 168
rhythm, 104
Roll-Up exercise, 77
Rolling Back exercise (Cadillac), 201
Rolling Down the Wall exercise, Wall Work (Magic Circle), 240-241
Rolling In and Out exercise (Barrels), 228
Rolling Like a Ball exercise, 80
    wobble-free rolls, 81
Rollover exercise, 122-123
rotator cuff muscles, 168
    infraspinatus, 168
    subscapularis, 168
    supraspinatus, 168
    teres minor, 168
Round Back, Reformer Stomach Massage Series, 191
rules for breathing, 41
    avoid holding breath, 42

avoid running on empty, 42
monitor breathing, 43-44
stop mouth-breathing, 43
vow to get more air, 42-43
Running exercise (Universal Reformer), 195

S

sacral vertebrae, 23
safety
    Cadillac, 199-200
    practicing Pilates during pregnancy, 13-14
    Wunda Chair, 213
Saw exercise, 84-85
scapula stabilization, 68-70
Scissors exercise, 140
    Barrels, 227
Scoop exercise (Navel to Spine), 62-63
    securing when doing sit-ups, 90
Seal exercise, 86
self-discipline, 6
sequence
sequence of exercises, 105-106, 122, 137-138
    Barrels, 224
    Cadillac, 200
    Magic Circle, 232-233
    Standing Arm Series, 170
    Universal Reformer, 185-186
    Wall Work, Magic Circle, 238
    Wunda Chair, 213
serratus anterior muscle, 28, 68, 168
services you plan to offer, teaching as a business, 262
Short Box Series (Universal Reformer), 192
    Fists in the Belly exercise, 192
    Flat Back exercise, 193
    Side Bend exercise, 194
Shoulder Bridge exercise, 110-111
    adding intensity with kicks, 124-125
shoulders
    muscles, 167
        deltoids, 168
        rotator cuff, 168
    posture, 24-25
Side Bend exercise, Reformer Short Box Series, 194

Side Kick Series (anticellulite solution for your bottom half), 152-160
  Beat-Beat Up, 155
  Beats on the Belly, 156
  Bicycle, 163-164
  Close the Hatch, 159
  Double-Leg Lift, 158
  Flutter Kicks, 160
  Grande Ronde de Jambe, 161-162
  Hot Potato, 161
  Inner Thigh Circles, 159
  Parallel Leg, 158
  Side Kicks, 154
  Side Passe, 155
  Small Circles, 157
  staying square, 153
Side Kicks exercise, as part of Side Kick Series, 154
Side Passe exercise, as part of Side Kick Series, 155
Side Stretch exercise, 176
Single-Leg Kick exercise, 97-98
Single-Leg Stretch exercise, 82
Sit in a Chair exercise, Wall Work (Magic Circle), 239-240
sit-ups, securing your scoop, 89-90
sitz bones, 70
Slide Down the Wall exercise, Wall Work (Magic Circle), 238
slumping posture, 23
  head positioning, 25
  kyphosis, 24
  shoulder positioning, 24-25
Small Barrel. *See* Spine Corrector
Small Circles exercise, as part of Side Kick Series, 157
spinal articulation, 65
spinal cord, 21
spine
  anatomy, 21-22
    discs, 21
    spinal cord, 21
    vertebrae, 21
  Barrels equipment, 222-229
    Arm Circles exercise, 229
    Backward Stretch exercise, 225
    Bicycle exercise, 227-228
    functions, 223
    Horseback exercise, 224
    Low Barrel exercises, 226
    Rolling In and Out exercise, 228
    Scissors exercise, 227
    sequence of exercises, 224

curves, 23
flexibility, Rollover exercise, 122-123
relaxation, Child's Pose, 99
Single-Kick exercise, 97-98
support, 28
  latissimus dorsi, 28
  rhomboids, 28
  serratus anterior, 28
  trapezius muscle, 28
Swan exercise, 95-97
Spine Corrector (Small Barrel equipment), cost, 222
Spine Stretch exercise, 84
  Wunda Chair, 218
Spine to Mat exercise (Anchor your Spine), 64
Spine Twist exercise, detoxifying your body, 125-126
springs
  Reformer, 182
  Wunda Chair, 213
stability
  hip, 70
  muscles, *transversus abdominal*, 58
  scapula, 70
  Shoulder Bridge exercise, 110-111
  trunk, 70
    Corkscrew exercise, 94-95
stacking your spine bone by bone, 22
stamina, increasing with proper breathing, 39
standardization, lack of in certification programs, 275
Standing Arm Series (arm exercises), 169
  Arm Circles exercise, 174-175
  Biceps Curls exercise, 170
  Boxing exercise, 171
  Chest Expansion exercise, 175
  Fly exercise, 172-173
  sequence, 170
  Side Stretch exercise, 176
  Zip-Up exercise, 173
Standing Arm Work (Magic Circle), 234
staying square, Side Kick Series, 153
sternocleidomastoid muscle, 167
Stomach Massage Series (Universal Reformer), 190
  Arm Circles, 192
  Arms Back, 191
  Round Back, 191

Straight-Leg Stretch, as part of Fives Series, 106
strategies for the teacher of Pilates, 249
strength of muscles, athletic performance, 15-16
Stretch with Pumping Arms exercise (Wunda Chair), 216
stretches
  Backward, Barrels equipment, 225
  Double Straight-Leg, as part of Fives Series, 107
  Double-Leg, 83
  Hamstring, 78-79
  Knee (Reformer), 194-195
  Side, 176
  Single-Leg, 82
  Spine, 84
    Wunda Chair exercise, 218
  Straight-Leg, as part of Fives Series, 106
  Tendon, Reformer Footwork Series, 187
subscapularis rotator cuff muscle, 168
supination, 184
support for the spine, 28
  latissimus dorsi, 28
  rhomboids, 28
  serratus anterior, 28
  trapezius muscle, 28
supraspinatus rotator cuff muscle, 168
Swan Dive exercise, adding intensity to the Swan, 138
Swan exercise, 95-97
  Wunda Chair, 216-217
sway back, 22
Swimming exercise, 112-113
symmetrical training, muscle imbalances, 59
synovial fluids, happy joints, 77

T

teaching, 246
  as a business
    attracting investors with a business plan, 260-261
    booking clients, 263
    choosing location, 265
    determining space needed, 264-265
    equipment costs, 258
    figuring potential profits, 263
    hiring teachers, 263

homebody versus gym body, 257-258
legalities, 258-260
marketing, 265-266
purchasing equipment, 266-267
services you plan to offer, 262
certification programs, 279
lack of standardization, 275
searching for programs, 273-275
time commitment, 272-273
commitment, 246, 254
dancers, 253-254
dealing with clients, 251
developing step-by-step progression, 251-252
hands-on training, 252
patience, 253
practicing KISS, 252
praise results, 253
designing custom programs, FIT (Frequency, Intensity, and Time), 249-251
desire, 256
emotional support system, 247
getting to know students, 247-248
listening to clients, 255
strategies for the teacher, 249
treatment of clients, 254
Teaser 1 exercise, 111-112
Teaser exercise, adding intensity to Teaser 1, 128
Tendon Stretch, Footwork Series (Reformer), 187
tensing the muscles, 166
accumulation of lactic acid, 166
upper trapezius, 166
teres minor rotator cuff muscle, 168
testimonies for Pilates method, 3-5
theory of opposition, 120-121
thermogenesis, 49
thinking body, 5-6
thinking yourself tall (posture), 30
thoracic vertebrae, 23
Time (part of FIT), 251
toxins, detoxifying your body with breathing, 37-38, 125-126

training, 46
awareness of body form, 61
conscious versus unconscious movement, 60-61
course levels, 274
Level I, 274
Level II, 274
Level III, 274
Level IV, 275
equipment costs, 258
guiding principles, 46
centering, 47
concentration, 46
control, 46, 92
controlled breathing, 48
maintain flow, 47, 103
precision, 47
homebody versus gym body, 257-258
metabolism, 48
thermogenesis, 49
plans, 50
symmetry, muscle imbalances, 59
transversus abdominis muscle, 29, 58
trapeze (Cadillac), 198
trapezius muscle, 28, 168
traps. *See trapezius* muscle
triceps muscles, 168
trunk stabilization, 70
Corkscrew exercise, 94-95
Twist exercise, 145-147

U

unconscious movement versus conscious, 60-61
Universal Reformer. *See* Reformer
upper back muscles, 167-168
arms
biceps, 168
triceps, 168
back
latissimus dorsi, 168
rhomboids, 168
serratus anterior, 168
trapezius, 168
chest
pectoralis major, 168
pectoralis minor, 168
shoulders
deltoids, 168
rotator cuff muscles, 168
upper Body De-Jiggle exercises (Magic Circle), Standing Arm Work, 234

V–W

"V" position, 74-75
Footwork Series (Reformer), 187
vertebra by vertebra movement, 22
vertebrae, 21
cervical, 23
coccygeal, 23
lumbar, 23
sacral, 23
thoracic, 23
visualization, 46
vow to get more air (breathing rule), 42-43

Wall Work (Magic Circle), 237-238
Rolling Down the Wall exercise, 240-241
sequence of exercises, 238
Sit in a Chair exercise, 239-240
Slide Down the Wall exercise, 238
Washer Woman exercise (Wunda Chair), 214
Web sites
wobble-free rolls (Rolling Like a Ball exercise), 81
Wunda Chair (equipment), 211-212
challenge, 213
cost, 212
functions, 212
Jackknife exercise, 217
Pike exercise, 214
safety, 213
sequence of exercises, 213
Spine Stretch exercise, 218
springs, 213
Stretch with Pumping Arms exercise, 216
Swan exercise, 216-217
Washer Woman exercise, 214

X–Z

Zip-Up exercise, 173

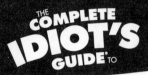
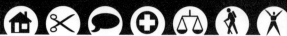